"*The Hiss of Hope* is a dramatic *catabasis*, a lived account of the journey we all face: hope hemmed by powerlessness, aspiration curbed by external forces. In those encounters, we lament our plight, and yet are summoned to find what meaning can be wrested from the descent. Oenning-Hodgson's book moves me to tears as I find courage and despair side by side, powerless allied with fierce independence, and through it all, both a model and a summons to ask ourselves, as Jung asked, 'what supports us when nothing supports us?' What sustains a sense of autonomy, dignity, and purpose when the old life has fallen away? The reader will share a journey with a woman of insight and courage, and be reminded of what we all have to draw upon when our appointment with life comes due."

James Hollis, Ph.D. is an author and Jungian Analyst in practice in Washington, D.C.

"There are many surprises on the journey Meredith Oenning-Hodgson shares in **The Hiss of Hope**. The tragedy and inevitable suffering associated with the illness, the onset of symptoms and the progressive disability associated with Parkinson's disease; these are woven seamlessly into the fabric of an intense human journey, exploring deep regions of the self, unraveling the meaning of significant developmental moments, reaching outward to explore intimate relationships with remarkable people in Meredith's world. Through all this is braided the ever-present specter of Parkinson's, relentlessly and mercilessly insisting on meeting Meredith's gaze in what becomes an essential intimate expression of autonomy. Revealed in the illumination of Meredith's self-reflection is an indomitable human spirit afire with deep psychological courage diving deep into the analytic depths of remarkably complex relationships developed with her illness, herself and those she loves. Truly, this is a worthwhile voyage."

J. Rowan Scott is a Clinical Professor of Psychiatry, teaching psychotherapy, family therapy and consciousness studies in the University of Alberta Department of Psychiatry. He has an interest in integrating the work of Complexity Science with the treatment of psychiatric syndromes.

D1287737

"My sister, Meredith, has written an amazing personal account of her journey struggling against, and *living with*, Parkinson's disease over twenty years. Parkinson's poses an especially difficult challenge, but everyone, if they don't get hit by a bus, get shot, or otherwise meet an early demise, will face their own suffering. We all lose physical control at some point; we can expect to deal with pain and with debilitating conditions (old age if nothing else). Meredith charts a pioneering journey into new ways to relate to the realities of our physical, mortal being. She finds—or better, creates—a pattern of relating to the painful oppositional forces of Parkinson's disease that transforms them into energies for growth, and can be applied in any relationship. It is a courageous journey through unavoidable suffering toward greater physical, psychological, and spiritual wellbeing. We all must find our own way; but *The Hiss of Hope,* one unique story of a trailblazing voyage, can also be a guide and inspiration— or at least point the way to new paths."

James P. Boggs, PhD Cultural Anthropologist

"Analytical psychology gives little consideration to chronic illnesses or physical impairment. On the other hand, published studies of physical disease or disability largely ignore psychological concerns. Only those who suffer an illness know how it feels; Meredith Oenning-Hodgson has the rare talent to enter into a deep dialogue with the illness, to let herself be changed by this uninvited lifelong guest, and to influence the guest in turn. Even more rare is her gift to recognize this process of the soul and to bring multiple literary sources to bear on this awareness: The personal becomes universally relevant. Meredith Oenning-Hodgson's elucidation of this connection makes *The Hiss of Hope* a treasure to be valued by those suffering a disease and by psychological and physical therapists. The book challenges all to take themselves, their souls, and their illness seriously and to encourage a dialectical relationship among them all."

Kathrin Asper, Dr. phil., Analyst, ISAPZurich

The *Hiss* of Hope

Galatea. From Isolde Ohlbaum, 2000, *Denn alle Lust will Ewigkeit*, Muenchen: Knesebeck. Used with permission of Isolde Ohlbaum. The figure on the cover metaphorically portrays the author when Parkinson's "freezes" her. Concurrently, the statue represents the mythical Galatea.

THE
HISS
OF
HOPE

A Voyage with Parkinson's
Toward an Intimate Autonomy

Meredith Oenning-Hodgson

CHIRON PUBLICATIONS • ASHEVILLE, NORTH CAROLINA

www.ChironPublications.com

Interior and cover design by Danijela Mijailovic
Printed primarily in the United States of America.

ISBN 978-1-63051-700-7 paperback
ISBN 978-1-63051-701-4 hardcover
ISBN 978-1-63051-702-1 electronic
ISBN 978-1-63051-703-8 limited edition paperback

Library of Congress Cataloging-in-Publication Data Pending

To all those whose lives have been dramatically interrupted by a force that compels them to restructure their worlds.

Notes for the Reader

Bd. is the German abbreviation for *Band* = Volume. Footnotes taken from a German source are noted as Bd.; footnotes taken from an English source are noted as CW = Collected Works.

Translations from English to German or German to English are my own, unless otherwise noted.

Acknowledgements

For the gift of this profession and patients who have enriched my heart and have challenged my mind, I am deeply grateful. There are so many, in Germany as well as in Canada and the USA, who have influenced me and whose stories I carry in me.

I am indebted to C. G. Jung and Wolfgang Giegerich, each for his pioneer spirit, the depth of thought, and the courage to express their revolutionary ideas. They have challenged and inspired me, and many others.

Anna. A *baby whisperer*, a nurse, my partner in this narrative of touching the space of the *hiss*, of searching around in the labyrinth of an *intimate autonomy* to arrive once again at where we began. But different. Anna's unbroken accompaniment, her unshakable presence of being, and her dedication to our process has been unparalleled. The depth of my gratitude knows no bounds.

John. My husband, who has been with me through nights and days of suffering under Parkinson's disease, whose music and humor I treasure, whose loyalty I commend, and without whose love and support I could not have written this book.

Anton. My son, whose letter ignites my search for the *with* and who accompanies me as a critic and, simultaneously, as an encourager.

The dragonfly. It has been the source of my writing and has mapped my transmutations. Its short but radiantly blazing life, its beauty, its transience, its mobility and kaleidoscope eyes that see "beyond," have guided and inspired me.

There are so many with whom I have shared the travails and thrills of writing this book, who have supported and encouraged me: my sister Jacqueline West; my brother Jim Boggs; Rosi Bambach and Melanie Higgins; Doro Jaekel-Ewald, Helga Wehmeyer, Vangie Bergum, Ray Benton-Evans, Janice Antonio, Vivienne Robertson, Rowan Scott, Frank Burman, Alex Fidyk, Stephanie Grabhorn. And many others. Thank you.

I also want to acknowledge and thank the four people who have been willing to be contacted for an endorsement or blurb: James Hollis, Katrin Asper, James Boggs, and Rowan Scott.

For Jennifer Fitzgerald, the general manager of Chiron Publications, for her help. I am grateful. Her patience, her midwifery, her encouragement, and her warmth have been exceptional. Thank you, Jennifer

And last, but certainly not least, I would like to express my gratitude to Eva Radford, who helped me put *The Hiss of Hope* in clean and clear form, and who has accompanied me and encouraged me to "get this book out there!"

Foreword
The Hiss of Hope:
Voyage with Parkinson's
into an Intimate Autonomy

It is a challenge to find words that can serve as a "foreword" to this book since the book itself takes us backward as well as forward, into and around, flying high and diving deep into an experience of living with the arrival of Parkinson's disease. As the book unveils this experience, we meet a depth of life and its relationship to death; we enter an experience that is profoundly held.

As a dedicated Jungian analyst, Meredith Oenning-Hodgson has created a book that is a unique portrait of a detailed analytic experience of battling with as well as relating to an unfathomably cruel illness, Parkinson's disease. Weaving her poetic, mythological, and literary mind, deeply rooted in philosophical reflections, into her analytic perspective that spans the oeuvre of Jung and its development through time up to the current extrapolations of Wolfgang Giegerich has been, and is, an ambitious—and remarkably healing—adventure. The totally original presentation in this book of her multileveled experience offers the reader a journey into and through gut-level and soulful anguish as well as remarkably well-portrayed personal transformation.

The author's experiences and reflections are presented in a truly creative way; they defy a simple, logical progression; they do not obey our familiar, well-organized chapter-by-chapter mode. Instead, she has chosen to introduce herself and her experiences in this book by allowing them to enter here, then there, at times biographically, at times poetically. She introduces herself and describes her experiences, adding reflections and amplifications as she proceeds. She progressively builds an environment that ultimately is paradoxically deeply integrated and that very intimately portrays her realities. Ultimately, the pieces about the psychoanalytic ground she is walking on come into perspective. Gradually, the philosophical and literary world she lives in comes into focus. All the while, the emergence of her capacity to wrestle with and ultimately form a relationship to the ever-present anguish of Parkinson's disease takes us, the reader, into an experience of emergent soul-strength that is deeply inspiring.

Meanwhile, for me, writing these words about her words is, in its own unique way, a particularly rich experience. I, too, am a Jungian analyst and I am thus the author's professional "sister"—as well as her biological/psychological sister. Though we have lived our adult lives geographically far apart, over the decades we have woven together a tender and profoundly essential relationship out of both remarkably fine but also very diverse and rough threads. It is truly a deep gift to have participated in the evolution of our relationship, a pattern of "intimate autonomy." It is with yet another layer of appreciation of her depth of being, which is so lyrically at play in this book, that I encourage you, the reader to dive in, swim with her—and watch your own breath as you read.

—Jacqueline West

Table of Contents

Foreword, Jacqueline West   11
Introduction   25

Part One   27
The parts   28
Structures and spaces   29
The hiss of hope   30
Intimacy and autonomy   31
Parkinson's and me   34
The hidden depth of structure   36
The alchemical nature of structure   39
Patterns   40
Our voyage   41
Intimate autonomy's anatomy   43
The quality of nothingness   45
Secrets of nothingness   47
Creativity   49
The play space   51
The house and me   53
Structures: Words, exoskeletons, scaffolds, and repetition compulsions   55
The word   56
Exoskeletons and the dragonfly   59
The house scaffold   60
Repetition compulsions   61
Intimate autonomy   62
Hope, no-hope, and their hiss   64

Part Two   67
Summaries   67
Now   67
Prologue   69
The molts (Latin: *mutare*, "to change")   70
Molt 16: Intimate autonomy's anatomy   73
Molt 15: "Formation, Transformation,/The Eternal Mind's Eternal Animation" 74
Molt 14: Anna   75

Molt 13: Alchemical moments and clinical vignettes of the voyage into an intimate autonomy   75
Molt 12: The dynamic dialectic of play—Galatea   77
Molt 11: The transmutation of the ice mirror   78
Molt 10: The dis-union   78
Molt 9: The dragonfly   79
Molt 8: The pitbull and the kitten—a two-in-one movement   80
Molt 7: The egg   80
Molt 6: Optimal oppositional friction   81
Molt 5: The dragonfly nymph   82
Molt 4: The pregnancy   83
Molt 3: The birth   83
Molt 2: The split   84
Molt 1: Anaclitic therapy   84
Final Molt: The dance of colors   85
The emergence into the adult phase   86
Epilogue   87

Part Three   91
Transmogrification   91
Molt 16: Intimate autonomy's anatomy   91
Fairy tale blueprints of an intimate autonomous relating pattern   97
The king of the birds   97
Florinda and Yoringal   99
Personal experiences of an intimate autonomy   101
Molt 15: "Formation, Transformation, Eternal Mind's Eternal Animation"   102
Molt 14: Anna   104
Molt 13: Alchemical moments and clinical vignettes of the voyage into an intimate autonomy   108
Alchemical moments   109
The paradox and beyond   111
Parkinson's and I   113
Anna and I   115
Vignettes from Anna's and my voyage   116
John and I   120
The dragonfly and I   121
Ahab and Moby Dick   121
The regressive space   122
A clinical vignette   124

Table of Contents

A child of light is born — 127
Molt 12: The dynamic dialectic of play—Galatea — 130
Galatea — 130
Upside-down play — 132
Molt 11: The transmutation of the ice mirror — 136
The movement — 138
The real — 139
Molt 10: The disunion — 142
The fractured union — 144
The white cat — 145
The narcissist — 148
Molt 9: The dragonfly — 149
My dance with the dragonfly: Peering into the looking glass — 150
The dragonfly and me — 150
Dreams — 155
Molt 8: The pitbull and the kitten: A two-in-one movement — 161
The pitbull — 162
Fractals — 165
The word — 167
The pitbull and the kitten — 168
Molt 7: The egg — 169
Chaos theory — 171
Anna's and my relating patterns — 173
The birth of the pitbull — 175
Molt 6: Optimal oppositional friction — 178
Molt 5: The dragonfly nymph — 189
Digesting the active imagination — 190
Anna's and my separation — 192
Molt 4: The pregnancy — 194
The placenta — 195
The good-enough mother scaffolding — 197
Introjection — 199
Real — 200
Pregnancy — 200
Molt 3: The birth — 201
Three transformational requisites for flying — 202
Molt 2: The split — 204
The regression — 205
The vertical split — 208
Isaac Newton, the scientific alchemist — 212
Molt 1: Anaclitic therapy — 216
Regression revisited — 216

The third space revisited   219
The third space   220
A personal account of anaclitic therapy   221
Anecdotes from our anaclitic therapy   229
Final Molt: The dance of colors   231
Red and white   232
The whiteness of the whale   235
The dragon fly   236
The narrative   237
Emergence into the adult phase   240
The dance   240
My dance into an intimate autonomy: a reflection of the dragonfly   243
A fugitive autonomy   248
The word   251
The hiss of hope (I)   252
Epilogue   253
Dragonfly eyes   253
My eyes   254
Repetition compulsion   257
Parkinson's disease   259
The centrality of me   261
The hiss of hope (II)   263

APPENDICES
Appendix A-1: T. S. Eliot, "Burnt Norton" from The Four Quartets (1935)   265
Appendix A-2: Hafez, "Every Child Has Known God"   267
Appendix A-3: Alfred Lord Tennyson, "The Two Voices"   267
Appendix A-4: W. H. Davies, "The Dragonfly"   268
Appendix A-5: Kahlil Gibran, "On Death"   269
Appendix A-6: Paul Celan, "Death Fugue"/"Todesfuge"   270
Appendix A-7: "East Coker," from The Four Quartets   273
Appendix A-8: T. S. Eliot, "A Game of Chess" and "Death by Water,"
from The Wasteland   274
Appendix A-9: Rainer Maria Rilke, Duino Elegies "The Eighth Elegy"/
"Die Achte Elegie"   275
Appendix A-10: William Butler Yeats, "The Second Coming"   276
Appendix A-11: Rainer Marie Rilke, "The First Elegy"/"Die Erste Elegie"   277
Appendix A-12: Alfred Lord Tennyson, "In Memorian," Section 45   278
Appendix A-13: Rainer Maria Rilke, "Archaic Torso of Apollo"/
"Archaischer Torso Apollos"   278

Figure: The vertical and horizontal splits   280

References   280
About the Author   288

Prologue

Eleven years ago, for my birthday, my son wrote me this letter:

Happy Birthday Mom,

The big 65! I know because you're always 30 years older than I am. Which means I've known you for 35 years now. I can't really say much about your first 30 years, but I CAN say your last 35 years have been chock full of hard work, lots of love, and invaluable wisdoms you have shared with me. Recognize and celebrate all these years today. You've had a prosperous, prolific, and peaceful life. Those all start with a 'p' and so does Parkinson's ... and that has been a new and important chapter. So, if there is one wish for your birthday, it is that you grow old 'with' Parkinson's, not in spite of it.

Happy Birthday.

Much love,

Anton

This book traces my journey during the last eight years, a journey to this state of *with* of Anton's birthday wish. What is this *with*? What does it look like? Or feel like? What is it not? This book traces sketches of labyrinthian lines: round ones, straight, curved, and wavy ones. There are periods, commas, exclamation points. But the process keeps going. There is no center reached. Not yet. But there is, however, a *with* won. This *with* I define as the dialectic dynamic of the relating pattern intrinsic to an intimate autonomy. It is the *hiss* of hope—a state between—and beyond the opposites of hope and no-hope. It is where I abide. For now.

In 1997, Parkinson's disease violently and invasively interrupts my life, both my personal and my professional life as a practicing psychoanalyst. From then on, everything takes place in a split world, a dualistic world, a world partitioned between a before and an after Parkinson's disease. For 20 years now, Parkinson's and I have been together. For the first few years, he is quite gentle with me, but soon he becomes violent, invasive, and demanding. I don't flee from him. I cannot. I do fight him. Or I freeze. Like the Snow Queen. Or often I feel like a statue—no, I *am* a statue. Like Galatea. Sometimes I sit—rigid for five hours. I have no choice. My spirit departs in disgust, as my body concedes to Parkinson's. And Parkinson's laughs with bitter scorn.

At the beginning of a love affair, one often says to the other, "Oh, I would so love to grow old with you." Often, it is not possible; the two do not make it. The *with* has long since dissolved into mist. Our beginning has not been a love affair—quite the opposite. But our relationship has not condensed into mere mist. At the present moment, we actually appreciate our togetherness, our state of an intimate autonomy. Sometimes I experience myself as being mostly auto-nomous. I move as if Parkinson's has receded out of my life. Then Parkinson's shocks me back into intimacy. Sometimes Parkinson's drifts off, and I forget that we will be together for the rest of my life. But there is a balance now, a dance wherein both of us can laugh at ourselves and at life. And at death.

Like *intimacy* and *autonomy*, the words *hope* and *no-hope* are opposites. If they are too separate, the words do not meet Anton's *with*. Nor if the opposites are too close. The two can become lost in a *folie a deux*, in an identification. Any two are in a space of paradox if they can be close and distant simultaneously and hold the tension. Their energies join while remaining separate; they connect and clash, yet neither disappears. Each is both intimate and autonomous.

This tension, this paradoxical energy, is of unfamiliar strength. The pressure of the clash between the two generates a new synthesis. This uncharted experience I've called the *hiss of hope*. It is a moment, an experience of not *doing* anything yourself; instead, something is happening to you. It is rare. An even deeper depth and higher summit as a result of paradoxical energy, is the unfamiliar *kairos* experience, an *out of time and structures* event. One becomes aware of life outside, or inside, the more common borders.

This leads to my use of the word *hiss* in the title of this book. The word—composed of letters—is a structural device. It serves as a containing form for the energy of the opposites of hope and no-hope when they can be close, but not too close, and maintain their differences while not being too far apart to dialogue. When the relationship between two is bedded in an intimate autonomy, a paradox, then the *hiss* happens.

Aside from the alliteration factor, the word *hiss* is not semantically interesting. It is a syntactical tool to convey the kinship, the intimacy, of alliteration with the difference, the autonomy, of its quality of presence. Hope and no-hope are conceptual; *hiss* is acoustically perceived. It has a sibilant liquidity that makes its presence known. This space demands its experience through the word *hiss*, a type of incarnated paradox, a "word made flesh."

I notice that when I am in this space between and beyond opposition, I can feel at the least a hint of wholeness, a balance, a corollary of an intimate autonomous relating pattern: a *with* evoked in my son's letter. The structural form of the paradox, a relating pattern that sparks the *hiss,* interweaves my son's *with* and the voyage, toward an intimate autonomy into the narrative of *The Hiss of Hope*. The *kairos* remains veiled in the mist of distant shores.

In this book I describe an eight-year voyage into a *with*, into what has become the underpinning structure for all my relationships, into an *intimate autonomy*. Intimacy is the implicit experience of being able to slide along the lines of a relating pattern that takes you gradually to a place of yielding to an *other,* and you know that in this process you will not lose yourself. To be *autonomous*, you slide also along the lines of the relating pattern but now you open yourself explicitly to vulnerability. You simply know that no matter what happens with such openness, you can cope with potential mental or physical assaults. The trajectories of this relating pattern are etched in my cells and are coagulated in my blood. I *am* now this pattern of relating.

The words *intimate autonomy* suggest a paradoxical relating. Is there such a thing as a paradoxical relationship with a disease? Does not a paradox itself assume the end of a thought? Can one think further than a paradox? Can one become more conscious?

In *The Hiss of Hope* I wrestle with the concept of an intimate autonomy, with the notion that the paradox constructs a gate, a form, a structure that opens to a space the mind cannot grasp, a state the eyes cannot see, nor the senses recognize. I use the tools of fairy tales, myths, active imagination, poetry, and prose to further illuminate this space. The constitutive blueprint of the process of an intimate autonomy unfolds along the line of the Hegelian principle of the dialectical thesis-antithesis and the inevitable synthesis (Houlgate, 2005). The synthesis is concomitantly the new thesis on another level. This process perpetuates itself: It is an autopoietic dance of life (Capra, 1996).

Both explicitly and implicitly, I feel held by a paradoxical scaffold of a flowing solidified softness. I feel guided by a source hitherto unknown. And I've learned to trust the dynamic process of the dance of the opposites and its self-birthing. Continually, new choreographies integral to an intimate autonomy are designed, and I am able to avoid the entanglement of Parkinson's expansionist behavior.

Parkinson's disease is a movement disorder. This book describes the gradual transmutation of this prime symptom into an increasingly *ordered* and uniform kinetic activity. There is now an overall symmetry between Parkinson's and me. It feels as if we are working together rather than in some kind of opposition to each other. I have learned a choreography that enables the once-upon-a-time movement dis-order to transform into movements that order themselves. I can now be with Parkinson's disease and—for the most part—we can move together: as one and as two, synchronized. In a weird yet welcome equality we order our movements. Like the *still dancing* of the dragonfly that conceptually for me has become what the Native Americans call a spirit animal, whose mutations define many of the paths taken by me to discover this pattern of relating, and whose wings can carry me to moments of physical and mental equilibrium (Eliot, 1935).[1] In Parkinson's and my relationship currently, there is structurally a rhythmic balance, no matter what the moment contains. And being together often awakens gratitude and warmth rather than the previous icy impact of anger, fear, or cutting disdain.

On the voyage to the *with* with Parkinson's disease, three accompany me, three who are willing and able to be still and to dance at the same time, together and privately. My husband, a retired geography professor, who is dedicated to this process—and to an *us*. The dragonfly whose mutations my body seems to adjust to in human form. And Anna. She is the pole. I dance around her, I dance with her, I dance against her, and I let myself be danced by her. Ultimately, it is the relating pattern of an intimate autonomy that dances all three of us.

I discover in the interpersonal relationship with Anna that intimacy does not deny access to autonomy. Nor does autonomy preclude intimacy. The new relating pattern has emitted some kind of data onto the more intrapsychic connection with Parkinson's, and it gradually begins to mirror Anna's and my relationship. Parkinson's and I morph into a viable couple, a twosome, bearing witness to unity and difference simultaneously.

It has been a voyage, sometimes falling into the waves and their turbulence, frequently riding high on the waves' crest, often being lulled into the rhythm of the water's soft and soothing undulation. Both Parkinson's and me. And Anna and me. For much of the time now Parkinson's leaves me alone. He does not insist on the previous entanglement—like the relating pattern between Ahab and Moby Dick.

---

[1] "…Except for the point, the still point, there would be no dance, and there is only the dance." The relevant portion of "Burnt Norton" is located in Appendix A-1.

Nor is he willing to separate, to dissolve and disappear into oceanic waters.

We all seem to have settled into intimately autonomous relationships. Including the unpredictable ocean and me. In general, the waters are calm and clear. I can swim, I can dive, and I can just tread water. Or I can do nothing. And wait.

The Hiss of Hope does not offer practical advice (Okun, 2015). It does not counsel and instruct how to feel like a "lucky man," Michael J. Fox's reaction to his Parkinsonian experiences (Fox, 2003). Nor does it take the reader to a space where the body becomes a "sinister stranger" (Friedman, 2017). Neither a cultural nor an anthropological/political concern is a foremost focus of this book. Rather, it suggests a structural, syntactical pattern of relating—not a personal exposition on love, feelings, and the individual emotional content of a relationship. This pattern, concomitantly, can be relevant for relationships of a more collective nature. Whether in a business, an environmental organization, or a committee on modern art, the structure of an intimate autonomous relating pattern can consciously be used as a coaching tool (Schenk, 2012).

My emphasis in *The Hiss of Hope* is on the role of the individual psyche. It is a narrative of a personal, individual voyage, a journey highlighting the transmutation of the structure of a relationship anchored in dualistic power battles to a relationship harboring the dynamic dialectical pattern of an intimate autonomy. It argues that the psyche is a neglected and often overlooked aspect of any physical illness; that a psychological frame of reference can open to spaces otherwise concealed or not considered. Understanding even a whisper of the patient's psyche can reveal a trigger of an illness; perhaps it can even disclose the source.

This is a relevant and perhaps a noteworthy book for anyone with a chronic disease such as Parkinson's. It will appeal especially to therapists, psychologists, and psychoanalysts and will be of value for all those who appreciate and enjoy being in relationships where autonomy is not lost and intimacy can be found. Recognizing the *hiss*, in its positioning itself beyond hope, and its opposite, no-hope, is a self-generating experience. The word *hiss*, like an orchestra conductor, regulates and coordinates oppositional combative energies, while gathering together its own sensual melodic chords of each letter. *Hiss* choreographs relating patterns structurally, vital to an intimate autonomy, and it loudly confirms the impact and the compliance of the request for a *with* from the birthday card of 11 years ago.

Introduction

I have written a chronicle of our journey into this unfamiliar landscape, into this territory of the "unity of unity and difference" (Giegerich, 1998). We discover new terrain that opens perspectives revealing previously untried trajectories.

Our voyage began in 2009. I stopped writing in 2015. Two years have passed. Currently, it is spring in the year 2017. Everyone is astounded that my physical limitations have been reduced to such an extent that this disease is at times hardly noticeable. I still have to be conscious of sudden enervation, of medication, of Parkinson's in general. But for the most part, due to nakedly exposing and opening psychological blockage, due to the recognition of psychic sources also generating physical symptoms, Parkinson's has waived his right to regard himself as an exclusively physical entity. He plays with the psyche now; they both share power and humbleness, and they dance together while remaining apart (Giegerich, 2010).

Currently, old patterns still haunt me but quickly recede into the haze of oceanic mists. The unusual dialectic of a paradox radiates into and onto—and has become the gestalt for—every other interconnection. It all happened like this:

Part One

The beginning. December 1996. I am in Santa Fe as usual for Christmas. I remember sitting together with my sister at the kitchen island. Writing a card?

All of sudden my hand wants to say something, and instead of expressing the desired word, it begins to flutter like a tiny bird that cannot yet fly. My sister and I laugh. Then I try again, and the writing flows as usual.

March 1997. I am back in Frankfurt. My hand refuses more and more often even to try to launch itself from the nest. Together with a colleague, a clinical psychologist, we decide to confer with a neurologist acquaintance of ours. On the way there, I remember saying, "*Gott*, I hope it isn't Parkinson's" (a disease I know nothing about).

In May 1997, in a small village on a wooded hill near Frankfurt am Main, the medical staff of an acclaimed Parkinson's clinic confirms the diagnosis of Parkinson's disease.

The diagnosis is not a fear of flying, but rather the intuitively perceived Parkinson's. Is it the same? Perhaps I am to learn to trust that the wings of the wind can carry me while in flight.

In June of that same year I had planned to get married. I know it is now impossible and decide to fly to Canada to tell him. Of course, the marriage is off. No man is going to be willing to let himself be burdened with Parkinson's in the house, in his life. I burst into tears when he immediately takes my hand and says, "In sickness and in health, 'til death do us part."

March 1999. I move to Canada after 32 years in Germany.

In 2009, Anna and I begin our voyage into an intimate autonomy. Anna flies from Frankfurt to Edmonton. In the beginning, she remains here for two months, then in 2013, she gradually begins to stay longer. In 2014, four months, two in the winter and two in the summer. In 2015, the same. My narrative stops here. My journey continues.

The process, the journey with myriad experiences, lines straight, slanted, and serpentine, with exclamation points, question marks, with commas, colons—sometimes a numerical biblical reference, sometimes a differentiation between hours and minutes, sometimes a syntactical introduction of things to come. Dashes. Few dots. Seldom is there a period, an ending.

The parts

Part One of *The Hiss of Hope* is the most challenging in the book. Just as thoughts have to be thought to come alive and music has to be played in order to be heard, this book can only come alive if you, dear reader, enter into a relationship with the words written: because most of the words in this part of the book are *thoughts' thoughts*. (I am indebted to Wolfgang Giegerich for his accompaniment and en-couragement in my efforts to experience his thoughts come alive!) But your task is now to listen for your own *irrational* music in these *rational* thoughts. If you can hear the notes, then you are ready to continue on to parts two and three. Claudio Abbado, the great conductor of Gustav Mahler's symphonies, who could hear each individual player while at the same time weaving the music into an organic whole, knew the moment of *being in the Hiss space*, where the individual and the collective come together: autonomously and intimately. Concurrently. So, please don't give up on the first part of this book. It's far easier to then sit back after experiencing thoughts' thoughts come to life, and then be able to sit back, relax, and listen to the music of parts 2 and 3. You can possibly catch the individual notes embedded in the whole.

Part One

Structures and spaces

"Thoughts need to be thought and in this way come to life, much like music needs to be played."
(Giegerich, 2010)

Before I begin, it is perhaps relevant to note my reasons for writing this book.

During the years I lived in Germany, I became enthralled with myriad aspects of German culture: their music, their differentiation between *Sie* and *Du*, and, most importantly, their literature. I dive into Rilke's elegies and soar with his "angels that terrify"; I recognize that Nathan is truly wise; I feel the Kafkaesque need—and failure—to change his life; and I am shocked by Borchert's: "there is no answer" (Borchert, 1947)[2] at the end of his drama *Draussen vor der Tuer*. Reading the poems of a more contemporary poet, Paul Celan[3], I weep. But the piece of German literature that I quite frankly fell in love with is Goethe's *Faust I & II*.

After being in Canada for a while, I feel compelled to make *Faust* more accessible to English-speaking people. There are but few in North America who have ever heard of *Faust*. I have taught *Faust* at the Jung Institute in Kuesnacht, Zürich, and am familiar with teaching both parts in German and in English.

So, I begin writing about *Faust* after a few months in Edmonton, and at the exact moment I begin writing about the conversation between Mephistopheles—disguised as Faust—and the Student

---

[2] German translation: "es gibt keine Antwort."

[3] Theodor Adorno of the Frankfurter Schule, who had proclaimed that there could be no poem after Auschwitz, writes: "Celan's poems want to speak of the most extreme horror through silence. Their truth content itself becomes negative. They imitate a language beneath the helpless language of human beings, indeed beneath all organic language: it is that of the dead speaking of stones and stars." Theodor W. Adorno (1970). Aesthetische theorie. In G. Adorno & R. Tiedemann (Eds.): Frankfurt am Main: Suhrkamp Verlag, p. 322.

regarding "the Word" (*das Wort*), I suddenly stop, and the thought comes swirling out of somewhere: This is exactly what Jung means with the Trickster archetype. And what Goethe expresses with Mephisto's introduction: "I am part of that energy, that always wants to do evil, and I always end up doing good" (*Faust* line 2016, trans. Trunz, 1966). And then, yet another thought comes whirling out of nowhere: I recall Jung's definition of God: "That's the word I use to describe any force which violently and without any sensitivity or concern interrupts my subjective plans, opinions or intentions. Anything that could care less what happens to me and turns my life upside down" (Jung, 1956-1961, p. 276, author's translation)[4]

Is Parkinson's an *evil* that is actually doing *good*?

And I feel torn away from *Faust* and begin writing *The Hiss of Hope*.

The hiss of hope

I hope. And I hope. I want to hope. I need to hope!

Slowly, gradually, I feel frustrated. After a period of concentrated effort, I unravel a possible cause: I am constantly propelling myself into the future! So, what happens if I do not hope? What is the opposite of hope? No-hope. Does that sink me into the past? It doesn't feel that way. Instead, no-hope rather violently discharges me into a no-time. An emptiness, a depression. A nothingness? Tension ripples throughout my body. The usual inevitable tension between opposites. Hope and no-hope are discordant. (Simultaneously, I recognize that opposites can spiral into a source of freedom from ego consciousness.)

While I sit and enjoy a surge of the soaring elation of intellectual gymnastics, I take a deep breath. Breathe in through the nose, hold it

---

[4] "Es ist das Wort, mit dem ich alles benenne, was meinen vorsaetzlichen Weg gewaltsam und ruecksichtlos durchkreuzt, alles, was meine subjektive Anschauungen, Plaene und Absichten umstuerzt und meinen Lebenslauf auf Gedeih und Verderb in andere Richtungen draengt."

until the count of five, and then breathe out through the mouth. That is the yogic method I know.

Something peculiar happens. I remember reading that past experiences integrate in present time, that this happens through bodily systems, and that consciousness is a process (Edelman, 2004, pp. 8, 115, 172). Consciousness is not a thing. These thoughts begin to float around in the saliva that has gathered during the count to five. The breath coagulates the memory of the *h* of the word *hope*. The breath also makes its way through the spaces between my teeth, and I hear multiple esses; I sense saliva gathering in my mouth. This physical process of sibilation crystallizes into the word *hiss*. Is *hiss* a child of the dialectical contradiction and friction of the opposites of hope and no-hope?

I am dislodged and involuntarily find myself vibrating in present time. The presence of the present encircles me. I feel there is not dualistic tension between *hiss* and hope as there is between hope and no-hope. I don't feel a compulsion to select one or the other. Nor do I experience an energetic fight/flight response. Hoping and *hissing* feel rather like a kind of dance, a kind of invitation to play with the fallout of the paradoxical energy of hope and no-hope. The *hiss* is also an invitation to sense the process itself and to become aware of the allure of movement inherent in paradoxical disharmony. The *hiss* of hope can derail fight/flight binary trajectories. *Hiss* moments can coax an intimate autonomy, whose paradoxical energy can in turn summon yet another *hiss*…

This repetitive process assumes the shape of a spiral, not of a circle. It is the syntax of an unfolding, a gradual transmutation; it is Jung's individuation (Jung, 1971, Bd. 16, para 442).

Intimacy and autonomy

I decide to attempt to relate to Parkinson's within this new pattern. I want a relationship that cultivates intimacy and simultaneously encourages autonomy. In spaces where present time prevails, where the pronounced physical structure of the word *hiss* commands attention, where the intimate autonomous relating pattern absorbs intimations of dualism, of the exclusive rightness of the one or of the other, of warring twos. I want a dance of paradox's subjective swirl escorting me from the two to a one, and back again...and forth again...and again. Until these opposites become a vessel in which "what was previously now one thing and now another floats vibrating, so that the painful suspension between opposites gradually changes into the bilateral activity of the point in the center" (Edinger, 1985, p. 143).[5] This point in the center is the fallout of the paradox. The point of the center is the *hiss*. And it is the beginning of a new spiral. This point in the center is autopoietic (self-birthing).

Parkinson's itself harbors a binary system of being on or of being off, and thereby sets up an internal dualistic dissension. Parkinson's renders me off, and my physical mobility is restricted. When I am on, I feel a freedom of movement. Often, I feel like a marble statue of Galatea, sometimes allied with death, the off phase, and then flipped into life, the on phase.

Parkinsonian rhythm is intrinsically oppositional, dualistic. The dance is mobility or immobility. This disease is known as a movement disorder. Unlike the *hiss* and the hope that can open a space, the *dis* denotes negation, invalidation. The *dis* in movement disorder touches a chord of irony, in that it deems movement—its very collaborator— incommensurable.

With Parkinson's disease as my partner, I decide to take a voyage to the initially jarring paradoxical motions of our intimate autonomy. Kinetic incongruity gradually transmutes into a measured compatibility, and Jung's point at the center can be—at least—intuited.

Intimacy can be experienced when I am able to lose ego control and yet know that I am not going to fall apart. Instead, I encounter a fluid, melodious, perhaps even a lyrical dimension of me. Autonomy is the part of this relating pattern that fosters a tender distance. It is not

---

[5] Edinger quotes from Jung's Mysterium Coniunctionis, CW, par. 296.

a separation. Autonomy is possible when I allow myself to be vulnerable in a relationship, when I can be defenseless, powerless. In addition, it is relevant to underscore that such an autonomy opens to empathy.

The cadence of the words *intimate autonomy*, the whiff of space between dualistic disorder, impels me to dance. Splashes of joy obviate an oppositional disparity in favor of mercurial liquidity. This underlying transmutation sets the tenor of the book.

The paradoxical distillation of this relating pattern, a core topic of my book, is a reflection of a learned dance, which has been the pivotal source of my relationship with a *good-enough mother*, Anna, and our experiences in an anaclitic therapy.[6] Anna's and my relating pattern has demanded a partial relinquishment of ego-control and a consciousness of the safety, the sanctuary, and the sustenance of intimate autonomy's initiation of a centripetal center that is a wellspring to further growth.

Leitmotifs throughout the book are: 1) the structure of an initial two, the *hiss* instead of the opposites of the hope and the no-hopes; for example of *hisses* and hopes, of Parkinson's and me, the ons and offs of the disease, of Anna and me, as well as Ahab and Moby Dick, and two fairy tale sketched twos; 2) the gradual transformation from the more separate and immobile twos into a dynamic dialectic, a fluid one, then both spill into "a syzygyial unity of the unity and difference of the opposites" (Geigerich, 2012, p. 307)[7]; 3) the transmutation of kaleidoscopic pieces in a dualistic fight/flight opposition to the dialectic of a dragonfly-like twirling caper, whose conceivable source is the poet's paradoxical dance at the "still point" (Eliot, 1943),[8] or Jung's bilateral point; and 4) the voyage to the *hiss* of an intimate autonomy.

---

[6] Anaclitic therapy is explained in detail in Molt 1. The term good-enough mother was coined by D. W. Winnicott and has become an iconic descriptive phrase for a mother who is not perfect but whose care of the infant is sufficiently nurturing.

[7] Syzygy: Twos that are in conjunction with each other and are simultaneously different. C.G. Jung uses the anima and the animus as a syzygy. It is not a "Third."

[8] The relevant portion of Eliot's poem "Burnt Norton," from which I quote the words still point, is located in Appendix A-1.

The Hiss of Hope is a chronicle of the choreography of time, space, movement, and of relationships; the dance of structures, of exoskeletons, and of repetition compulsions; a written record of Parkinson's disease and our journey into an intimate autonomy.

Parkinson's and me

Some time ago I decided to stop trying to find meaning in the fact that I have Parkinson's. I decided to stop trying to establish a cause-and-effect chain for the attacks that leave me immobile. I decide to cut the closeness, the intimacy, between us, and I decide to structure an autonomous life for us both.

This resolution has failed, of course. One cannot decide to live without an illness that insists on becoming part of one's life. I do want to change something, nonetheless. I am determined to do something about the relating pattern that exists between the disease and me.

This thought dances in me and, simultaneously, in Parkinson's as it has become my partner. But thoughts become peripheral when Parkinson's physical dualistic movement disorder begins its singular dance. Parkinson's migrates to my interior and attacks. This incursion from the inside catches me. It is as if a sour and toxic entity has ambushed and invaded. It feels as if an interior octopus sadistically uses its arms to grab from the inside. These tentacles pull on every inch of me; they interlock tighter and tighter. I become immobilized. I cannot do anything but hold the tension. And I wait. My voice is pressed to a soft, barely utterable sound. My breath is left with what feels like tiny narrow pipes through which it can flow. This condition lasts usually for three to five hours. Then, all of a sudden, the octopus finds other fish in the sea, and I feel once again freed from Parkinson's disease.

In this present moment, while I can still taste and know Parkinson's sensuously, physically, and recognize the second it demands its narcissistic claim to my body, I decide to consciously accede to this involuntary intimacy. And at the same time that I yield to the too-closeness, ironically perhaps, I hope to establish more of a conceptual distance between us, more of an autonomy for both Parkinson's and for me. Perhaps the mere thought about Parkinson's and our potential mutual autonomy can think this relating pattern into existence. Perhaps the thought's thought opens up a space somewhere between the brain and the body, a space ignited by its oppositional moment of an intimacy that is quickened by the discordant notion of autonomy, a space that bonds and animates the relating pattern of an intimate autonomy. Quite like when my architect father emphasized that the structural design of a building is not the significant aspect, but rather it is the spaces within. This accords the structure of a building—like the structure of a thought—a living presence, a womb-like containment birthing itself into life (Giegerich, 2012, pp. 107-108).[9]

Suddenly, I know I have to write. And I have to write about relation-ship. Not the usual emphasis on the meaning or feelings associated with a partnership, but on the structure of such a connection: I am going to be concerned with patterns of relating, with the living syntax of a relationship rather than with the everyday linguistic semantics of what our relationship feels like. With the pattern of an intimate autonomy I want to forfeit the search for meaning in favor of climbing inside a structural configuration, a syntactical entity like the strings of words or

---

[9] "If it needs to transcend itself in order to come into its own, then this means that it exists as its own self-sublation. Its sublation does not lead out and away, but deeper into itself… we have to realize that it would transcend and sublate itself all by itself provided that one would allow it to be experienced thinkingly."

Wolfgang Giegerich has "thrown the spear" of psychology further. With his courage and creativity he dares to be poised on the cusp of a new consciousness. In 1913, C. G. Jung's critique of the Freudian school of psychoanalysis opened similar new doors of per-ception and offered insights new for that time. Just as Jungian psychotherapists at that time took Jung's critique of Freudian psychoanalysis seriously, currently we can be open to the insights offered by Giegerich. The emotional and the intellectual premises among Jun-gian therapists can then perhaps become even more consciously perceived. Or—as in my case—Giegerich's "doors" can open to new spaces. From Giegerich's book What is Soul? I want to underline ideas relevant to our voyage. On page 46, Giegerich defines soul as ac-tuosity, "full of movement, life, abounding in action." He emphasizes, "There is not such a thing as soul." Later on pages 56-57 he elucidates that the soul "only comes into being when two fundamentally separate things come together and interact…the soul cannot be pre-sent in isolation…it is only as the between." On page 60, Giegerich writes that the soul "by losing itself, it finds itself, comes home to itself." Like the spaces of the architect. Or the movement of the soul endemic to Goethe's Higher Health. Like an intimate autonomy?

of symbols like geometrical forms, and become part of this meta language unfolding or revealing its own space, of its birthing itself.

The hidden depth of structure

"Thought is not an ego activity.... The I is of course needed, in fact indispensible, but only as the place where the...seeds can do their own ripening"
(Giegerich, 2010, Vol. 10, p. 19).

One needs to move beyond the "voice of the intellect" to the formulation of "an as yet uncreated system of mystical rationality"
(Heinz, 1985, p.70). [10]

Three examples of the conscious use of structure, or form, or syntax, either bequeathing space or arising out of space can help to clarify my emphasis on structure. (Throughout the book, I will be using *structure, form,* and *syntax* interchangeably, and likewise the words *space, content,* and *semantics.*) One can perhaps maintain that form is the apex of content; that syntax is the culmination of semantics; that structure births space—as my father always emphatically pointed out to anyone listening. Three templates of the employment of patterns, the tracks of repetitive structures to generate a relationship, can elucidate my emphasis on the voyage to an intimate autonomy, to a form that choreographs itself out of its rhythmic dance of closeness and distance. These are but a few examples of the often-overlooked pre-eminence of structure to content, or of form to substance, or of syntax to semantics.

Meditative practitioners repeat a mantra in order to slide along a syntactic structure. One repeats the words again and again without

---

[10] Cited in Jones, J. W. (2002). Terror and transformation: The ambiguity of religion in psychoanalytic perspective. Routledge: London.

concern or interest in content or the semantics of the word(s) repeated. Rather, the meditator slithers down the forms of the letters, the words, to reach a cusp of consciousness otherwise hidden. One can land in a space hitherto unknown, a space perhaps even revealing an unfamiliar part of oneself. A new self-relationship is unveiled. Some are led to a new consciousness connecting with the collective. To a world-connection hitherto averted. Perhaps by an Ahabian narcissism, an inability to see beyond oneself to an other, an imprisonment in one's own oneness. The world on Ahab's projection screen is a relationship only of a one. He sees the white whale, Moby Dick, as himself.

The hidden depth of structure can open to the viewer of a painting. The artist uses geometrical forms as structural invitations to discover secret spaces hidden from the common eye. He fills these spaces with color, often with red, and encourages the viewer to slide on the geometrical structures, and thereby slither through the color content of red on the canvas into a new relating pattern, both for the viewer and for the artist. Using the color and the light—and the forms—as "instruments," the artist explains, both she and the viewer can fall through the painting into a shared truth. And "the seeds can do their own ripening." This can be a shift into an intimate autonomy.[11]

One last, yet significant, example of a structural path to a depth otherwise unseen and a relating pattern otherwise hidden is in the pictures in the book, *Das Magische Auge/The Magic Eye* (2002/2004).[12]

---

[11] Mark Rothko himself describes these blocks of various colors as possessing their own life force, their own "breath of life." For Rothko, light and color are "merely an instrument." The abstract, the pure form, enhances "clarity" and "destroys illusion and reveals truth." Rothko does not use words to express anything about his paintings. He explains: "Silence is so accurate." When people "break down and weep" before them, this proves that he expresses "un-seen" human emotions, which are only perceived when one slides through the visible color content. The New Yorker, April 12, 2010, pp 80-81.

[12] This interest began in 1959, when Dr. Bela Julesz began researching depth perception. By 1991, computer programmers and artists came together and created a new form of art, a new way of viewing the world: the magic eye. In addition to the scientific and artistic interest, eye specialists have claimed that these exercises improve the eye's vision and strength. The patterns, the colors (as instruments), the structures and the networking of all of these enable the viewer to "see" beyond what others can see.

Computer programs containing algorithms generate pictures of repetitive patterns and structures. The challenge for the viewer is to slide past the picture presented to be able to see either a 3-D image or a coded sketch, both something totally unexpected. The instructions suggest that one should look through the lines and the dots in the picture to perceive what is concealed behind, or beyond, the obscure structural foreground.

The viewer's eyes seem to assume qualities similar to those of a dragonfly, whose eyes seem to be opened to sight. Their eyes do not assume the usual subjective task of seeing, but rather, they yield to being led by insights.

"Their [dragonfly] eyes are made up of 28,000 individual units. Each of these tiny facets faces a different direction and each produces a tiny image. The insect's brain puts all of these tiny images together to form a picture, much as we do with the dots on televisions and computer screens. More than 80% of their brain is devoted to analyzing visual information." (Oenning-Hodgson, 2009, p. 50) How the brain functions to enable the dragonfly to spot prey from as far away as 40 yards remains a mystery. Their ability to turn their heads almost completely around so that they can see below as well as above contributes to their spin through time: Dragonflies are ancient insects. They flew around when the dinosaurs ruled the world. The dinosaurs disappeared, but the dragonflies are still here.

Perhaps the dragonfly is able to be close to its environment without an entanglement. Perhaps it is able to maintain a tender separation from its environment at the same time and thus fly through space and time by riding the wind. An intimately autonomous relating pattern. How these seemingly vulnerable tiny creatures whose multi-faceted eyes dance with the brain and can turn on the 28,000 units and then transmute them to one picture remains yet a mystery to any systematic investigation. Perhaps their secret is the ability to look out with their singular insight and abide in the structural depth of an intimate autonomous relationship with themselves and with the world.

Part One

The alchemical nature of structure

I want to witness a structure's unveiling, its reinventing of itself by revealing itself spatially, without any manipulation or suggestive semantical seduction or augmentation. Indeed, the structure "dissolves itself in its own water" and thereby comes home to itself (Edinger, 1985, p. 1). [13] A transformation of matter. Embedded and quickened in this

---

[13] Perhaps an additional example of the "hidden depth of structure"—or of something dissolving in its own water—would be the role, the structural significance, of an orchestra conductor. With his baton he shepherds each member of the orchestra. The eyes of each individual musician follow the movement of this small narrow stick, its speed and its passion. With such a conductor as the recently deceased Claudio Abbado each individual player feels part of a whole, a 'one' and simultaneously concentrating on his own notes, the musician is swept up into an intimate autonomy. All this is due to the depth of the structure revealing itself from Abbado's beguiling wand.
Edinger writes:

> The process of psychotherapy, when it goes at all deep, sets into motion profound and mysterious happenings. It is very easy for both patient and therapist to lose their way. This is why narrow and inadequate theories of the psyche are clung to so desperately—at least they provide some sense of orientation. If we are not to submit psychic phenomena to the Procrustean bed of a preconceived theory, we must seek the categories for understanding the psyche within the psyche itself. An old alchemical dictum says, Dissolve the matter in its own water. (Edinger, 1985, p. 1)

This is what we do when we try to understand the process of psychotherapy in terms of alchemy.

The notion of interiority reflects the alchemical process of "dissolving in its own water." Giegerich writes:

> Psychology is the discipline of interiority. But this interiority is not in me, not in you, not in anybody, also not in the depth of any thing out there. It is in its (psychology's) own Notion itself, which, as we said before, is not the notion of something, but its own Notion of itself. Psychology has to allow itself to relentlessly fall into the thought that it is and use the depth of this thought as its mirror for reflecting whatever its subjects in each case might be. The soul or interiority of its objects is not in the objects themselves. It is in its, psychology's, own Notion, in the internal infinity of its absolute-negative interiorization or the internal infinity of its mirror. But within the 'subjectivity' of its own Notion, it has the objectivity of reality (in the sense of Wirklichkeit, not Realitat). (1985, p. 97)

> "The true inner is defined as that whose interiority has, in a revolutionary reversal, surrounded the very notion of 'outside', 'margin', or 'border' and internalized it into itself. The inner is thus what has the outer truly within and not outside of itself. Only this self-contradictory, 'crazy' relation is what constitutes interiority…." (Giegerich, 2010, p. 147)

39

transformation of matter is the process of alchemy, the medieval forerunner of chemistry. Psychologically, alchemy's anatomy can be viewed as a blueprint of life's journey from birth to maturity. And back and forth, and forth and back. Alchemy outlines paths—or structures, trajectories—to follow in order to attain consciousness, to reach a maturity potentially available to us as sentient beings. The cryptic alchemical symbols, diagrams, and textual imagery of alchemical works typically map potential passageways from an infant's identity with primal substance or dark matter (*nigredo*) to a strengthened consciousness of the more autonomous form of individual maturity. This is the gold (*rubedo*), the goal, of an alchemical journey: from the black of primal awareness to the red of conscious life. Transmutation of lead into gold is presented as an analogy for personal transmutation, purification, and perfection. Alchemically threaded throughout this process is the rhythm of a circular dance of opposites, of *dissolatio* and *coagulatio*.

This ancient wisdom reveals a dynamic uroboric form and function of knowing, a circular model, a *perpetuum mobile* energy. Endemic to this process of consciousness is the emphasis on *with*—a two, a relationship. Implicit in the word *consciousness* itself are the etymological Latin roots *con*, "with" or "together," and *scio*, "to know." Hidden in this rather hermetic—or cryptic—language—or, for our purposes, we could employ the word *structure*—are patterns of relating, patterns like an intimate autonomy—that encourage and underlie health. Secrets to help me live with Parkinson's disease.

Patterns

The seminal seed of structure's hidden depth is its inherent promise of patterns. Patterns are crucial to the understanding of living form. Indeed, it is said that in order to understand life, we must first understand patterns. To comprehend a pattern, recognition of relational structures is necessary. Patterns are relationship. "What connects the crab to the lobster and the orchid to the primrose and all four of them to me?" the anthropologist asks (Capra, 1966, p. 173). Once we have relational structures, we can be concerned about their patterns of relating, or of networking. The crucial word is *feedback*. Structures have to do with quantity, while patterns involve quality, the ephemeral connection, the relationship connection: a hidden depth.

The pattern of an intimate autonomy, the structure of this relationship with its hidden promise of life's quickening inevitability, has become the blueprint choreographing my relationship with Parkinson's. The flutter of movement hidden in this structural simplicity can be a relating pattern for any twos. A possible worldwide cultural revisioning. I can conceive of the twos—or the many—dissolving "in their own water" to a dialectic attunement of a one, to a changeable, to a more liquid—a more alive—relating pattern.

I want to experience Parkinson's and me not only as individual, separate, and warring twos, but I would like to sense our *hidden* one: a unity, a one, capable of sliding out again to a two. And back again to the one ad infinitum. The consciousness of the probable inevitability of this flow, of the structural liquidity of life itself governing my relating pattern with Parkinson's helps me to be present in the caught, the *off*, the marble statue phases. While immobilized, while feeling one with Parkinson's offness, I can gather units of meditative curiosity and wait to be *on* again. By now I can recognize patterns, tiny cues, faint structural shudders, byproducts of the liquidity of the oppositional ons and offs that signal freedom. I can anticipate the joy of being released from this physical imprisonment; I can anticipate the joy of movement, of melting, and of being *on* again. And I can taste the elation once again to be able to enjoy the experience of autonomy and smell the delight that I do not always have, to experience being the victim, being a mere object at the mercy of Parkinson's.

Our voyage

We are going on a voyage. The water guarantees movement, a structural covenant of oceanic currents. I want to suggest a relating pattern with Parkinson's that renders the dualism of the ons and offs as not necessarily only oppositional and fixed. Indeed, I want to suggest

THE HISS OF HOPE

that the puzzling structure of an intimate autonomy can quicken movement instead of the more common conviction that the two paradoxical words are semantically logically inconsistent and incommensurable, and are therefore static. The friction of any paradoxical twos can instigate a dialogue that can liquefy the twos into a one that can create a structural trajectory, a path that facilitates the flow back and forth. And forth and back. The linear course of a dualistic relating pattern gradually morphs into a more sinuous shape. Ultimately, there remains a fallout, an unfolding structural unknown, a *hiss* or kairos moment.

While on this voyage, the undertow of oceanic currents can wrest us down to dangerous depths, the waves can toss us up to harrowing heights. With both experiences, Parkinson's and I are off, we are out of control and at the mercy of dualistic forces. Back and forth and forth and back...we are still boomeranged between these opposites.

There is a third possibility. We are on, on top of the oceanic waters; here I am more in control of my life. Yet at the same time I am at the mercy of nature. Here Parkinson's and I gradually slide into an intimate autonomy. The oceanic waters can attain an optimal oppositional rhythm that contains the back and forth of the ons and the offs. My body trusts itself to be carried by these waters. Is an alchemical pulse signaling potential transformative change? The waves rise and they fall, they undulate, they dialogue. We are intimately rocked by the waves, while autonomously I can even play with the often overwhelming and inexorable rapidly changing currents. I float in and out of the waves. In this intimate autonomous relating pattern, I splash drops of oceanic waters wherever and whenever I want to, and I often laugh. Sometimes—now more often than before this voyage—the water drops mirror my smiles. And they do smile back, but with a smirk: I am warned of these same drops potentially transmuting to tears. Of hope dissolving into its *hiss*.

There are moments in this third space that hint of Goethe's higher health. The German poet and author reminds us that everything foreign and false is stripped away through suffering, and we can then open to the joy of *renunciation (Entsagung)* (Goethe, 1821/2012).[14]

---

[14] Goethe's Wilhelm Meister's Years of Travel, or, The Renunciants 1795-1821 (Wilhelm Meis-

Similarly, the English psychoanalyst and pediatrician D.W. Winnicott emphasized the opposites of good and bad health, and the transformative potential of an optimal oppositional trajectory to a true health when "healthy people can play about with psychosis...and know that we are poor indeed if we are only sane" (Davis & Wallbridge, 1981).

Intimate autonomy's anatomy

How does our voyage accommodate the contradictory undertow, the currents of a paradoxical relating pattern of being firmly self-sufficient and simultaneously closely attached? How does a pattern of relating evolve? Why is this pattern pertinent to our voyage? What is an intimate autonomy: its structure, pattern, and its network? And what is the structural base of an intimate autonomy's relating pattern?

To reiterate, the moments in this pattern, the key forces, that centripetally hold everything together are: 1) intimacy that is anchored on the ability to give of oneself without losing oneself; and 2) autonomy that is based on the navigability of vulnerability. These are the structural

---

ters Wanderjahre 1795-1821) is an example of growth through suffering. For Goethe, the concept of oppositional attunement (an intimate autonomy) is a "red thread" throughout his life. The dictum in his famous poem "Holy Yearning" (Heilige Sehnsucht), the axiom "die and become" (stirb und werde) is but one example. Dying, e.g., a qualified ego death, is a form of regression, a space opening to potential transformation. An illness, for example, or a psychic wound, can cause such an experience of dying—or of regression. It is often a shove in this direction. An optimal oppositional attunement or a balanced relating pattern with an illness can be a becoming, an opportunity toward a transformation, toward a "higher health (hoehere Gesundheit). The opposition between health and illness becomes attuned.

Conceptually, "health" is something different than freedom from suffering and illness. Goethe's years of physical suffering, of psychic depression, were opportunities for him to become aware of a Lebenskunst, to get to know the "art of living." The most important ingredient in life is to be open to change, to transformation, to new developments and attitudes.

Faust's famous words reiterate and summarize Goethe's means of attaining the attunement necessary for his higher health (hoerere Gesundheit): [unless otherwise noted, it will be my translations for the Goethe works] "formation, transformation/Eternal mind's eternal animation" (Gestaltung, Umgestaltung/Des ewigen Sinnes ewige Unterhaltung) (Faust II, lines 6286-6287).

underpinnings, the visceral anatomy, of an intimate autonomy. These are the cadences, the pulse of the structure, the pattern, and the network.

The structure ("substance, matter, quantity" (Capra, 1996, p. 158.): The structure of a system is the physical embodiment of its pattern. The relationship structure of the system of an intimate autonomy has two common trajectories: one outer, the interpersonal; and one inner, the intrapsychic. Each is concerned with the relating pattern of the I and the Other—or, in clinical terms, of the ego and its relationship objects. The interpersonal is the outer embodiment of this structure; for example, a relating pattern between my husband and me, or between my ego (the I) and a disease like Parkinson's (the Other). The embodiment inside is the relating between the ego (the I) and the Other (the intrapsychic Other; for example, images, anxiety, depression, or the potential disease like Parkinson's). The structure of the relating pattern of an ego and an illness can be viewed as both interpersonal and intrapsychic.

The structural system of either/or of an I and the Other, be these two involved either interpersonally or intrapsychically, is familiar and unambiguous. But the words *intimate autonomy* pose a problem: These words cancel each other out. What can be so impelling about words whose structures, whose syntactical patterns of relating, culminate in an empty nonsense? Most people can probably grasp being concerned with intimacy or—for that matter—with autonomy, but to feel the need to devote one's rare and valued time to the structure of a contradiction? With the emptiness of a nothingness? Why would one do this? Is there an answer?

The pattern: "form, order, quality" (Capra, 1996): The pattern, the organization of any system, is its truth, its core, its personal spirit, its soul, which is the energy of its life's process. For example, the pattern of an oak tree is in its acorn, the pattern of a human is hidden in a fertilized egg nestled in the mother's womb. The pattern is autopoietic, the pattern is the process, the living pulse of unfolding the organization; each component is a network of connections, of relationships. But what is the pattern, the core, the soul of our paradoxical intimate autonomy, of an empty nothingness?

The network: "We each exist in an eternal moment that…contains everything that came before and everything that will come, linked together in a complex feedback loop." (Robertson, 2009, p. 65)

Separation is an illusion. The world is a collection, a network of natural phenomena that is fundamentally interconnected and inter-dependent. The function of each component is to participate in the production or transformation of other components. Hidden in the structural relating pattern of this living web, the spaces for relationship lie in wait. These alchemical empty nothingness spaces provide the hidden depth necessary for each revelation of a structure's own truth having dissolved itself in "its own water." Anatomically, they are wombs waiting for life *in potentia*. Psychologically, these are spaces of regression, spaces sponsoring reorganization, rebirthing.

Patterns of relating are living forms. The physicist knows that "all living systems are networks of smaller components, and the web of life as a whole is a multilayered structure of connections nesting within other living webs—networks within networks." (Capra, 1996, p. 209) The emptiness of nothing spaces between the latticework of the webbing can be quickened by the networking.

The inevitability of connection is given by the structure of the networking; that is, each structure activates another structure. The prefix, *con*, of *connection*, a primal etymological wellspring that promises a *with*, confirms the pattern, the structure, and the network's functions.

In a living web, an intimately autonomous relating pattern is the adequate anatomical arrangement. Entanglement of the strands or split-off structures of a network break the web itself, and any processing relating pattern is lost.

The quality of nothingness

The structure, the pattern, and the network. Their syntax would seem to lend itself more readily to a quantitative, rather than qualitative, categorical cluster, and as such is mathematically measurable. The rational, logical connections soothe.

The qualitative nature—indeed, the relating pattern of a paradox—of an intimate autonomy can be frightening. Indeed, the irrational space of nothingness does not soothe.

The contradiction endemic to the paradox of an intimate autonomy—or to any paradoxical system, for that matter—creates a vacuum, a zero, a nothingness. There is no quantity that verifies reality or that offers an experience of support, of confirmation. It can be felt as a defeat for the ego. The ego loses control. It cannot assume its usual role of manipulating reality. Any attempt to use the zero of the paradox reinforces insecurity. Add or subtract a zero to a paradox and nothing happens. Multiply by zero and everything disappears. So, what is the significance, what is the sense of the structure, the pattern, or even the networking of our intimate autonomy? My father, who claimed that the spaces—the zeros—yielded by architectural design were the most important, pointed out, in addition, that the structures of the corners in these spaces can be designed to increase a patterned energy flow. "No right angles," he said. Imagine a house with the emphasis and concentration placed on zeros and on imagined energy. A house whose essence is nonmeasurable, a house you might want to live in, but a house whose substance is mathematically, rationally, not even there. Yet such a house stands!

The nothingness of the paradoxical intimate autonomy does offer something, however. The emptiness of this space opens the possibility of movement. (Parkinson's vibrates upon hearing this! Parkinson's has never liked the label of movement disorder!) The zeros can comprise networking curves that encourage energy flow. We can slide, we can play. And we can wait and curiously observe qualitative depths and potential quantitative entities born of movement and energy.

Part One

Secrets of nothingness

During my training at the C. G. Jung Institute in Zurich, a story circulated about one of Jung's patients:

A female patient brings a dream to Jung, a dream that shocks and disturbs her. In the dream, she is at the bottom of a deep well. Desperation and terror overwhelm her when she contemplates remaining stuck there. Anxiety lends her ego the strength to begin an ascent, an attempt to climb up and out of her imprisonment. She begins to search for bricks that could have ledges to hold on to with her hands and then to put her feet on. Time passes. She does in fact manage to climb up the brick walls of the well. From her scraped fingers, her grasping hands, even through her socks from her clinging feet, blood can be seen dripping down the walls she has clung to. Finally, after much time and effort she reaches the top. She pulls herself up with her last bit of energy and strength and peers over the edge of the well. Delighted to see Jung himself, with a faint and exhausted voice, she cries, "Jung, Dr. Jung, please help me!" She sees Jung turn towards her. He smiles. She is filled with hope and returns his smile. Dr. Jung comes to the edge of the well, looks deeply into her eyes, and then he pushes her down into the well from whence she came.

When I first hear this story, I am shocked and once again I wonder about this direction of psychology for me. I ponder on the terror triggered by the descent into the well, I ponder on the smile and Jung's subsequent betrayal. Much later, after comparable experiences of my own, I comprehend the structural impact of the downward thrust into the well. It is yet an additional example of the potential birth of form from the fecundity of the *non-egoic* space of nothingness. (For me, clinically, it becomes a shove into a deepened regression.)

Similarly, when I first hear C. G. Jung's answer to a question about knowing God from a reporter writing for *Good Housekeeping* magazine, I feel angry and perplexed. What could Jung's answer have to do with knowing God? A few days before Jung's death, the reporter asks Jung to define his notions of God. "To this day God is the name by which I designate all things which cross my willful path violently and recklessly,

47

THE HISS OF HOPE

all things which upset my subjective views, plans and intentions and change the course of my life for better or worse," Jung explains (Jung, 1961).[15] This is a rather unusual definition of God, and I often either have to smile or scream when I think about Parkinson's having the audacity to claim such a holy incarnation. For this disease has certainly interrupted my life. And has changed the course of my life. I often feel pushed into the well. Again and again. Unable to tap my usual ego-strength, I fall into the nothingness at the bottom. Or is it the top? Or the middle? Or is it just space? Or is it a me and a not-me? A place of truth?

There are other examples of the potential fertility of nothingness. I know this now. Nothingness is. And I do begin to comprehend the well story and Jung's definition of God. If I were to begin to play, the notion comes to mind: "There is not nothing in this space."

So, the questions remain: How do we get to the bottom of the well? How do we begin? Is there a beginning?

For the alchemist, the prime matter, or the *prima material,* is found at the bottom of the well. This is the one basic substance underlying all others. It is the basis for any transformational process. I think the *nigredo* is enfolded in the nothingness. Or the nothingness is enfolded in the *nigredo.*

> This Matter lies before the eyes of us all; everybody sees it, touches it, loves it, but knows it not…and is found every-where…our Matter has as many names as there are things in the world; that is why the foolish know it not… As concerns the Matter, it is, and contains within itself all that is needed (Waite, cited in Edinger, 1985, p. 11).

One can also cite the *prima materia* or simplistic structure of a Japanese garden as an example of relative nothingness: this rather stark, succinct, crisp scene of various-sized rocks placed together in an organized pattern. No vegetation, no green, the starkness of colorlessness. Being in a Japanese garden always feels cold to me. I want to

---

[15] Jung wrote this definition in a letter in 1959.

leave. But I often don't. I sit down on one of the large stones. I sit. I wait. But for what? It is not measurable. Yet I often feel a depth and a fullness unexpected in such austere simplicity. Unforeseen in the naked form.

I think of yet an additional example of the full emptiness of structure in a theological quotation, a paradoxical nonsense, yet the words entice us to play: "Of God we know nothing. But this ignorance is the ignorance of God." (Boesel & Keller, 2010, p. 2)

Creativity

A play with words. The paradox. Confessions of the artist: "Art is a lie that makes you know the Truth" suggests a hidden secret of nothing-ness, a secret transformative space (Picasso, 1923, pp. 270-271).

Our words, intimate autonomy, lie. How can one be intimate when she is autonomous? How can one be autonomous and at the same time be intimately related? There is no movement in either of the two words, no slack, no room even between the words to maneuver. The paradox lies. Each is a one. The two words are physically together yet they have nothing to say to each other. Indeed, they contradict each other. There is a movement disorder between them; that is, one could surmise that there is no movement between them. There is perhaps no communication.

Empirical science's rationality and our irrational paradox of intimate autonomy are incommensurable. Yet the possibility is opened for the ego to yield its exclusive tyranny, to withdraw and to wait, curious and expectant. It is easy to construe the opposites of irrationality and rationality to be dualistic. And to be static. If each opposite, however, "dissolves itself in its own water," if each of the two opens to its secret, if each internalizes and touches its own form, there is movement, movement in a one as well as in a two. Each is alive. The ego can consciously make an effort to establish communication between itself and the alive nothingness it faces. It can dialogue, it can dance, it can play. In any case, there is communication between quantitative and qualitative perspectives (Heisenberg, 1967).[16] Indeed, "playing with the fecundity of nothingness" invites an opportunity to allow oneself to enter naked—with less need to control—a space of relative emptiness. Such a space promises nothing. But it often unveils hidden truths that belie inert opposition.

Unless the two begin to play, each with itself as well as with each other, unless they can move into an oppositional attunement, into the structure, an interpersonal as well as an intrapsychic quantitative structure, there can be no qualitative pattern of relating. When readers respond with frustration and with anger at the abandonment felt with a paradox, the poet encourages them to play with the riddles or mysteries hidden in the folds of these contradictory words (Trunz, 1986, p. 464).

A moment of attunement can be experienced in a movement of play. The net begins working, the slide back and forth between the two words, and their conceptual birth of a one can crystallize. This is the moment when the lie begets truth. This is the moment when art can birth itself.

Truth is for me a conscious personal experience of nothingness and emptiness, and of some egolessness: I notice that I do not dissolve,

---

[16] Werner Heisenberg, the physicist and rational scientist, reminds us: "Even today we can learn from Goethe that we should not let everything else atrophy in favor of the one organ of rational analysis; that it is a matter, rather of seizing upon reality with all the organs that are given to us, and trusting that this reality will also reflect the essence of things, the 'one, the good and the true.' Goethe's way of science offers science a means to find a way to allow the natural world to present itself in a way by which it could speak if it were able." This text was taken from a lecture that Heisenberg gave to a conference on Goethe, May 21, 1967. (Wir werden von Goethe auch heute noch lernen können, dass wir nicht zugunsten des einen Organs, der rationalen Analyse, alle andern verkümmern lassen dürfen; dass es vielmehr darauf ankommt, mit allen Organen, die uns gegeben sind, die Wirklichkeit zu ergreifen und sich darauf zu verlassen, dass diese Wirklichkeit dann auch das Wesentliche, das «Eine, Gute, Wahre» spiegelt. Hoffen wir, dass dies der Zukunft besser gelingt, als es unserer Zeit, als es meiner Zeit, als es meiner Generation gelungen ist.) (Dieser Text war Vorlage für einen Vortrag, den Werner Heisenberg auf der Hauptversammlung der Goethe-Gesellschaft in Weimar am 21. Mai 1967 gehalten hat.)
See Seamon D. (1987). Goethe's approach to the natural world in implications for environmental theory and education in humanistic geography prospects and problems. In D. Levy and M. Samuels, Eds. Chicago: Maargufa: pp. 238-250. See also Bortoff H. (1996). The wholeness of nature: Goethe's way toward a science of conscious participation in nature. Herndon, VA: Lindesvarne Books.

I do not fall apart, I encounter. I encounter a core, a truth intrapsychically as well as interpersonally, I meet something other. The dance of the twos and the one begins. We whirl. We twirl. We dance as a two and are also a one.

And then I know that I'm not going to fall to pieces if I fall apart, if my ego lets go. As already emphasized, intimacy is possible when egos do not jam the connection and insist on defending against vulnerability. Vulnerability opens to a portal accessing autonomy. Only when I feel able to be vulnerable can I truly be autonomous. My need then translates into the freedom to enjoy. And only then is it possible to be both intimate and autonomous and to play with the paradox of this relating pattern. Or with any paradox. Or to thinkingly send the paradox into its own interiority.

The motion, the notion, the energy of the paradoxical pattern is quickened through contradiction; the energy is chaotic, it is a *perpetuum mobile* of electric opposites rubbing against each other. Every now and then the friction sparks and lights up a space, a space visible to those who can glimpse into the liminality of life and death, into the transient pulse of life itself. And perhaps death itself. It is a moment of relative egolessness, of nothingness, and of truth.

The play space

The play space is a third space. Or a fourth space. Or a fifth space. Its position in between is pivotal. It is an in-between-space. An interface between. This space is not even a thing; it *is* not. There is ideally a nanosecond when autonomy is not separate, not static, not dry, when intimacy is not entanglement, when autonomy and intimacy touch and then retreat from each other, when this movement vibrates, the two touch and spark, the in-between-space opens; it is the space of the *hiss*.

Nestled between the flowing twos and the interiorized ones there are openings where horizontal and vertical energies cross. A fire is kindled. Sparks fly. And if the consciousness of the artist is intimately present, yet autonomously open, some thing can be created. It is what the Greeks call a *kairos* moment. Such a moment is the Transfiguration of Jesus: "and his face did shine as the sun, and his raiment was white as the light...a bright cloud overshadowed them: and behold a voice out of the cloud, which said: This is my beloved son...hear ye him" (Matthew 17:2-5). This is the potential moment of creativity.

If this moment passes, if the voice is not heard, if there is no moment when opposites quicken, if the opposites are too far away from each other, or if they are too close to each other, there lingers a sense of dullness, a feeling of flatness. Or at the least, a sense of frustration.

For me, if the ons and the offs of Parkinson's catapult me from one to the other without centripetal energies pulling them together, then I can fall into a nothingness...and I fall through. I am not even at the bottom of the well. Indeed...there is no bottom.

A haunting depiction is offered by D. W. Winnicott, who expresses the experiences one can face if opposites remain static, if they stay unrelated. If there is no movement. If the opposites do not play with each other. If an in-between space and creative consciousness do not touch. Winnicott refers to this state as being in a space where "trust in the environment" evaporates and the atmosphere becomes inundating feelings of general anxiety, an "unthinkable anxiety [which is akin] to the threat of annihilation" (Davis & Wallbridge, 1981, p. 46).

I read these words. My breath becomes scarce. I experience myself disappearing. If I can hold the single solitary movement of my breath as a guarantee of life, if I can slide into the terror, then I can perhaps consciously gasp and inhale the movements of nothingness. Consciously, I recognize an opportunity to let go, to allow myself to slide into the terror, to test the potential dynamic inherent in nothingness. And perhaps to allow a reorganization of early trauma experienced by the tiny infant with strawberry-blonde hair.

I sense eyes that see me, breath that, like wind, blows through me, that touches me...such experiences transmute this terrified not-me back to also-me. The state of me and not-me...this nanosecond...if my ego can contain it, offers me creativity *in potentia*. I am in an intimate autonomy with myself. I am alive.

Movement, or the lack of movement, sets the script for any narrative of the play, or the third space. This space is conducive to feelings of trust as well as to experiences of terror. The linguistic structure most in character with this space is the paradox. A point, a simple point, but whose complexity, whose energy derived from the self-contradiction of oppositional dynamics, burns a hole that can open to the mysteries of creativity—or this point can be a slide down to Winnicott's unthinkable anxiety (Jung, 1984, Bd. 14/1, para. 41, pp. 69-70).[17]

The structure of the paradox, the pattern, the network, can take us to the cusp of a new consciousness. If you first let yourself slide into an intimacy with your ego and look inside, and then try to extricate yourself from this exclusive ego-connection, you can leap—or slide—into nothingness and can allow curiosity and a qualitative third space of play to impel you further and further. You can slide along the boundaries of a new landscape of a you and a not-you. The pattern, like our paradox of intimate autonomy, is a network of the mysterious; it is a sphinx-riddle with a grin, a smirk, because there is no answer. There is, however, a space to play. Or to dance. And without your ego being the agent, to create.

The house and me

"Come dance with me
Come dance!" [18]
(Hafez, 1320–1389)

My father was an architect and engineer. Growing up, my brother, my sister, and I were generously exposed to the singularly authentic houses

---

[17] This point is identical to the scintella...the spark of the soul...the light embedded in nature, the lumen naturae…. ("Der Punkt ist identisch mit der scintella...dem Seelenfunk...das lumen naturae….")

[18] The full text of Hafez's poem "Every Child has Known God" is located in Appendix A-2. In Thus Spoke Zarathustra, Prologue, Part Five, Nietzsche wrote, "You must have chaos within you to give birth to a dancing star."

designed by the famed architects Bruce Goff and Frank Lloyd Wright. We grew up in the house my father planned, designed and—with the help of his university students—constructed for us. When I was 10 years old, I watched them first construct a scaffold of wooden planks and iron poles, which then was sacrificed when the house was autonomous enough to stand on its own. The scaffold on the outside was the necessary containment, the indispensable provision for the birthing of the house.

I discover later that this house has been a major source of my sense of space, structure, and beauty. This house has also proven to be my blueprint for a vital relating pattern between man and nature, instead of man's feeble yet consistent need either to identify with nature and remain stuck in the intimacy of participation mystique, or later to be too distant from nature, to manipulate, to use her and bend her to his will. Or to submit to her will. This house of ours offers yet another choice: We have experienced that our house enters into a third pattern of relating to nature, a play space, a relating pattern of intimate autonomy, a pattern desperately needed in our twenty-first century. Nature's water, her rivers and streams, are threatened; her bees are close to becoming extinct. Throughout history, nature's invitation to us has remained a reflection of the inherent dynamic of a paradoxical pattern: She has said, "Come dance with me, come dance."

I hear the words of the 14th-century Persian poet, Hafez, when I open and allow memories of our house to unfold. The first, the foremost, the most alive recollection is sitting in front of my father's aesthetically sculptured copper hood over the fireplace: a V-shaped sheet of copper reaching up into the heavens through a glass sky-light. Throughout the years, the copper moved and danced with each fire we lit; with each flame the copper seemed to come alive and to swirl into a multitude of yet hidden colors. This dynamic dance between nature and man, the fire, the copper, the glass, and the sky has coagulated in my blood; its pattern of intimate autonomous relating has been etched in my cells; the sound of the wood *hissing* and snapping when entangled with a flame cues my heartbeat, and the whiff of sizzling, breaking, and smoldering wood still tickles my nose.

Copper is Aphrodite's metal; the dance of relationships is her dance. This book, *The Hiss of Hope*, is about her dance, about our dance, about the flames, the pain, and the years it takes to hold the intimacy of the increasingly vibrant and varied colors of relating patterns, and at the same time retain an autonomy, an individual development and an individual morphology (form and structure). Maturity in both the intimacy and in the autonomy blooms and opens; it occludes an "unripening into a bud" (Davis & Wallbridge, 1981, p. 8).

Structures: Words, exoskeletons, scaffolds, and repetition compulsions

"Formation, transformation, The Eternal Mind's eternal animation..." (*Faust II*, Oenning-Hodgson, Trans., lines 6277, 6278)[19]

Words, scaffolds, exoskeletons, and repetition compulsions are all structural net-workings endemic to transmutation. The scaffold, the initial outer frame necessary to construct the inner house, eventually loses its function and is sacrificed. The exoskeleton of the dragonfly provides protection for the larva until it molts. The exoskeleton is forfeited. My own inner repetition compulsions, the defensively protective structures, can be dissolved and internalized when vulnerability is contained, autonomy is gained, and intimacy is retained. Between the inner and the outer there seems to be an interfacing double-sided mirror that from its third-space positioning reflects and quickens outside scaffolds and exoskeletons while effecting an inner repetition compulsion. Reflective networking!

---

[19] My translation from the German: "Gestaltung, Umgestaltung,/ Des ewigen Sinnes ewige Unterhaltung."

The word[20]

Mephistopheles: For the most part—trust in the word!…
Student: But the word has to hint at a concept.…
Mephistopheles: But when a concept is missing,
Then a word can be swiftly found,
With words one can fight and disagree.
With words construct a system with glee.
On words one must swiftly believe,
The word demands that one take heed.
(*Faust,* Oenning-Hodgson, Trans., lines 1989-2000)

This book is a scaffold of words, a scaffold initiating the plan, the sketching, the designing, and the construction of our relating pattern. Our scaffold employs narrative and expressions from the 19th century of Herman Melville's *Moby Dick*. It emphasizes Ahab's relating pattern with the whale as a contrast to Anna's and my pattern of relating.

The word as an outside scaffold can open to an inside quality, that is, a rarely perceived aspect of itself. The word does breathe. Syntactically, the word can resound and reflect out of its interiorized, intrapsychic primordial depth. The poet claims the ability to hear the ancient embedded music, to feel its vibrating chords, and to smell its resonating roots, permeating time century after century (Hauptmann, 1862-1946, quoted in Campbell, 1959, p. 5).[21] The rims of each letter can open, and thousands of years cascade out of each reverberation. The echo touches a substance and resounds in matter.

---

[20] Mephistopheles: Im ganzen—haltet euch am Worte!…/Schueler: Doch ein Begriff muss bei dem Worte sein.…/Mephistopheles: Dann eben wo Begriffe fehlen,/Da stellt sich ein Wort zur rechten Zeit sich ein/,Mit Worten laesst sich trefflich streiten/Mit Worten ein System bereiten/.An Worten laesst sich trefflich glauben,/Von einem laesst sich kein Jota rauben.

[21] Gerhart Hauptmann (my translation): Poetry revivifies each word and evokes an echo of its primordial origin. ("Dichten heisst, hinter Worten das Urwort aufklingen zu lassen.")

As one of the crucial strands of the network, I want to emphasize and clarify the singularly important role of the word.

In the course of my being held together, first contained by structural repetition compulsive defenses long embedded, but then eventually evolving into my own molting maturation, and ultimately my emergence into the adult phase, the word's function has been to serve as a scaffold that often conceals and hides. My feelings, emotions, and personal thoughts have undergone transmutations, but most importantly, the word now does not have to serve as a protective structure for me. In an intimate autonomy, the word and I are both intimately involved and autonomously independent. The word's syntactical capacity holds sentences and paragraphs and constructs the form of written documentation in general. Words that question and do not answer leave spaces open. The word's scaffolding commitments on the outside as a prime singular entity can dissolve when it looks inside itself. Here creativity begins. Interiorized, it exposes its own truth and its vulnerability. The word becomes a quality of presence birthing itself. It can unveil its own endemic structure, its pattern, and its truth.

The word is pregnant with its own etymological origin, with ancient enigmatic melodies resounding through the centuries, with cadenced leaps into foreign heights and depths, and with utterances and physical tones hitherto relegated to the animal kingdom. We cannot always hear it.

Between scaffolding energies and its affinity with the wings of the dragonfly (*gefluegelte Worte* /words with wings"; idiomatic expressions) —and its subjective playing with my thoughts—the word assumes an invaluable role as an entity exemplifying intimate autonomy in motion. With me and with others—as well as with itself—the word assumes an intimate role while remaining singularly autonomous to its own syntactical significance. The word functions as a double-sided mirror. At the same time, it is a window to the inside and to the outside. It is a vehicle of movement. (If only my wings—or my words—could just take off on their own. If they could at least first fly about autonomously, before the intimacy of my ego-bound Puritan interference begins to swarm and retrench their flight. Or—perhaps even better—if they could just take off together with the dragonfly!)

In time the hermetic wings of the dragonfly, together with their dance with the word, both playing together with my thoughts, and my thought's thoughts, my images of the house, and of course, the steady accompaniment of Anna and our third space in our anaclitic therapy, bring forth The Hiss of Hope.[22]

My relationship with the word is highlighted throughout this book. The house designed by my father is likewise a trajectory that conveys and reflects the interconnection of the net. Equally syntactically abstracted and simultaneously foundational are my relationship with Anna and the anaclitic therapy, and my journey with the dragonfly. I have touched on these topics already, but their significance warrants a more in-depth account. I want to allocate to each a short descriptive account of their importance for me as well as for the voyage in general.

---

[22] To access the soul of an animal, an insect in my case, one does not "do" anything. It just happens. As does consciousness, often. It is part of the network. Perhaps growing up with the cultural heritage of the American Indian and their experience that humans and animals inhabit the physical world together and that therefore they must also inhabit the spirit world together, opened me for my experience of receiving the dragonfly [see my article "Illness as an Illusion of Misfortune" (2009)]. Or perhaps it was having read Phillip Pullman's Golden Compass series, in which a guillotine can separate the spirit animal (daemon) from the human and extract life energy or joie de vivre from the spirit animal. Or Carlos Castaneda's series in the 1960s, which contributed to my cultural and personal knowing of spirit animals.

In many Native American cultures, the vision quests are a turning point in life, a rite of passage, marking the transition between childhood and full acceptance into society as an adult. A traditional vision quest consists of a person spending four days and nights secluded in nature. They are to forgo sleep and food. The Lakota Sioux name for this quest is hembleciya, "crying for a dream." In a Big Dream the spirit animal is seen. Along the same lines, shaman practitioners receive a certain spirit animal, or power animal, as a guide. There are four types of guides: messenger, life, journey, and/or shadow guides. My dragonfly belongs to all of these, perhaps most clearly that of the journey guide. This spirit animal's gift is to come to you when a decision has to be made, when you are at a fork on the road of life and do not know which path to take. This power guide remains at your side until the journey is complete.

All this and more contributed to the dragonfly seeking me out to become my spirit animal and my recognition of its significance for me. We, the dragonfly and I, are in a relating pattern of an intimate autonomy. The dragonfly is my scaffold both physically and psychically, and perhaps my being his?

The word *dragonfly* as well as the actual presence of this insect had remained remote to me until, like Parkinson's, the dragonfly demanded a place of prominence in my life. And then… "An inner impulse rent the veil/Of his old husk: from head to tail." [23]

Exoskeletons and the dragonfly

Perhaps due to its role as my spirit animal, this insect enters my life like Parkinson's disease. It invades my house even though the walls, windows, and doors are all shut (Oenning-Hodgson, 2009, pp. 37-54). The journey into a distanced closeness is depicted in the pattern of interpersonal relating with Anna, but also both interpersonally and intrapsychically with the dragonfly. The dragonfly's mutational development, its shedding of exoskeletons, approximates the process of our house's scaffold being dismantled and my dispossession of repetition compulsive structures. The plan, the design, and the construction of the dragonfly and its metamorphoses reflect my journey depicted in *The Hiss of Hope*. The relationship between this insect and me reveals the pattern between a human and a spirit animal of any variety, provided the relationship avers the quality of presence due such a connection. This pattern of relating in Native American culture between a First Nations man and his spirit animal is most often a quintessential example of the paradox inherent in our unusually close yet distant intimate autonomy.

These cardinal threads network throughout *The Hiss of Hope*: the dragonfly, the word, the house, Anna, and the anaclitic therapy, this paradox's immanent animating energy. And the *hiss*, the pheno-menological synthesis between the notions of hope and no-hope. Words narrate the process of the intimate autonomous relating pattern between Anna and me as well as my liminal, seminal experience with

---

[23] The relevant portion of Tennyson's poem, The Two Voices (1833) is located in Appendix A-3.

the "king of flies" (Davies, 1928),[24] with the dragonfly, this "living flash of light" (Tennyson, 1833).[25]

The house scaffold

And our house? The house has molted, and the scaffold lies liquid, gradually bleeding into the earth. The house is standing strong. Various outer and inner structures have recognized a certain innate ability to bend, to emanate out from their constructed surfaces into intimate autonomous patterns of relating. There are but few right angles. The only feature yet incomplete is the glass in the window frames. These open spaces are like eyes that do not see. Our eyes take in particles of light, bending and refracting them, turning them into electric impulses, and then sending these to the brain. We actually see with our brains. Perhaps when the glass is in and the windows begin to dance with light, perhaps they will see in a manner foreign to us yet nonetheless contribute to a certain flow of energy in and out of the house. Perhaps the windows contribute to a consciousness, an awareness of a dynamic relating pattern, an intimate autonomous relationship between inside and outside, a dance that a house without these eyes would not be able to do. Through these eye windows the opposites melt into a fluid dance of light and electricity.

On the outside, landscaping is not in any manner planned, nor designed, nor constructed. On the inside, however, there is a towering blue spruce. The tree stands in the middle, in an open-roofed atrial space around which the house is built. The house seems to breathe and to be fed by a weird heart-like palpable energy emanating from the tree's ancient roots. These umbilical-like structures are partially visible and otherwise deeply, firmly embedded in the earth. Typically, my father's plan has been to design and to construct the house around this tree, bestowing on it an honor typical of his relating pattern with nature: a

---

[24] The relevant portion of Davies' poem "The Dragonfly," is located in Appendix A-4.
[25] The relevant portion of Tennyson's poem "The Two Voices" is located in Appendix A-3.

pattern of interlocking independence, an interwoven closeness and distance. The spruce is majestic, her branches reach out to the west, to the east, to the north and the south; they stretch up to the heavens and bend with the snow and with the rain down to the earth, where the roots assume their function of integrating the many with the one. The silver blue needles are the veins of the winged tree branches. I listen to hear the words the wind breathes out through the tips of the spruce needles.

My eyes can look through the empty window frames and be the glass that reflects a not-me back to myself. I am the glass that provides a protective yet transparent interface between the inner and the outer worlds. Like skin. A third space. A space between.

I remember hearing that Jung has recommended that we must remain in the storm in the valley while at the same time observing everything from the top of the mountain. I can intimately accompany myself, the closeness, the feelings. At the same time, from the back of my eyes, from a greater distance I can simultaneously, autonomously observe while I watch. And I would know that reflectively, inside me, Parkinson's disease is doing the same.

Any vestige of outside scaffolding is invisible; it is as if the structural containment had never been.

Repetition compulsions

Sigmund Freud's use of the concept of *repetition compulsion* (*Wiederholungszwang*) was articulated for the first time in the article of 1914, *"Erinnern, Wiederholen und Durcharbeiten"* ("Remembering, Repeating and Working Through"). Here, he notes how the patient does not *remember* anything of what he has forgotten and repressed, he *acts* it out, without, of course, knowing that he is repeating it. ... For instance, the patient does not say that he remembers that he used to be defiant and critical toward his parents' authority; instead, he behaves in that way to the doctor. (Freud, 1914)[26]

---

[26] Sigmund Freud uncovered what is now known as the repetition compulsion. Four main

I have come to recognize that this is one of Freud's most significant discoveries. Correspondingly, the structure of a repetition compulsion is central to analytic work; that is, its recognition, and the discernment of its echo. Only then can reorganization be possible. Indeed, only then can this inner structural scaffold "dissolve itself in its own water." Only then can the patient discover and feel her own truth. Only then can there be "formation, transformation/ eternal mind's eternal animation."

Clinically, my most unbendable repetition compulsion is the firmly entrenched and desperate need to maintain ego-control. With this compulsive structural scaffold in place, an intimate autonomy is challenged by the closeness of intimacy and the vulnerability of autonomy.

Intimate autonomy

I have danced while journeying with Parkinson's disease since the diagnosis in 1997, for 20 years now. My pivotal partners on this voyage are Parkinson's; the waters of the unconscious; Anna, my German collaborator in the anaclitic therapy;[27] my generous and caring husband; and the gracious gift of my spirit animal, the dragonfly. Ahab and the white whale's accompaniment reverberate as a constant oppositional force that shields and hides instead of shedding, exposing, and opening. Their presence provides a constant cautionary reminder to cultivate the relating pattern of our intimate autonomy. Ahab's identification with Moby Dick, a too-close relating pattern, stifles any

---

features occurred to him:
1) It originates from a traumatic experience.
2) The repetition compulsion is structural. The content differs at the varied stages in life.
3) The repetition compulsion is unconscious.
4) Words are not available because there is no memory of the traumatic event. The words are dissociated, unintegrated. Without words, thinking is not possible. So the path of discovery leads along observing repetitive structural behavior, thought, or affect.

[27] See Molt 1 for a detailed depiction of anaclitic therapy.

flow and suffocates any transformational growth. There is only a one. A two disappears, lost in the projective identification.

My common way of relating has changed from one of the usual fight/flight dualistic pattern to playing with a newly uncovered intimate autonomy, an optimal oppositional consensus, a qualitative unity possible only in the truth-processing dissonance of a dialectic paradox. I've noted that an intimacy encourages attachment while autonomy fosters vulnerability. Assuming the strength to withstand vulnerability, and to have the grace to dance with the anxiety of intimacy, I recognize that the *hiss* of hope requires the necessity of sovereignty and conscious boundaries. Attending this voyage, of course, have been the snowflakes of winters in Edmonton, the sunshine of July, and the rhythms of life. And of death.

These reorganizations do not just happen with the appearance of Cinderella's good fairy and her magic wand. They have been the result of learning and practicing this new dance pattern, and of being willing to cruise on the capricious waves of oceanic waters with little ego control. It has been a cruise ultimately teaching the art of giving oneself up to the dance itself as well as to the dance partner without losing oneself, a water ballet in which the structure of the physical movements dissolves into itself. Interiorized, these configurations and their fluctuations open a space where the ego is fundamentally a tourist, and this opening fills with the "inner mystery and inner infinity" of the truth, or the soul of an intimate autonomy (Giegerich, 1998, pp. 54, 57, 59).[28]

I listen for words conveyed by the wind, or to words whispering through the viaduct of my breath. (Both are perhaps transported by the hermetic breezes integral to the winged "flashes of light" emitted by the windows of the house as well as by the living dragonflies and the ghosts of dragonflies already passed.) I cannot seem to evade a refreshing rush of air harboring a hidden meaning to be guessed at. Or

---

[28] A paradox. Giegerich writes: "The soul is the spark that is ignited…the soul cannot be present in isolation.… It is the nature of the soul…it is the dialectic of interiority and out-wardization, the dialectic of life and death.… It is both at once, their contradiction" (pp. 54, 57, 59).

often I encounter an optimal oppositional friction that leaves a paradoxical open-endedness, a hovering question without an answer. The dances with Parkinson's and even with Anna at times have rendered me feeling helpless and victimized but have also allowed me at times to be at home in my well-known repetition compulsion of feeling in control. The structure of learning how to dance, to slide from one opposite to the other, to allow myself to actually become slippery and less in control, less in need of ego-leadership, has opened new worlds, alternative spaces, and moments of unused consciousness. I have become acquainted with my body being held on the water rather than being victimized by the undertow or the high waves. These new experiences, and the culminating energizing friction of the restructured relating pattern, a relationship of the increased vulnerability of a strengthened autonomy and its oppositional yet mirrored intimacy, seem to have birthed a new core, a core of a purring centripetal force and centrifugal strength.

The strategic structural finesse of this dance, this dance of scaffolds, of exoskeletons, of repetition compulsions, their early shielding and then their sacrificial sheddings and openings to a new autonomy, often to a second birth, is the fulcrum of the voyage (Tennyson, 1850).[29]

Hope, no-hope, and their hiss

The dance continues and leaves traces of its movement around and among hope, no-hope, and their *hiss*. Intertwined dynamically with the other myriad threads of the net, I can hear the faint chords of hope carried by the wind into the future. No-hope screams from the past. The echo of *hiss* resounds, bounces from strand to strand, and, remembering Ahab's last words to the whale, *hiss* affirms its presence with the words: "I spit my last breath at thee" (Melville, 1847/1967, p. 468). *Hiss* lassoes hope and laughingly reminds it not to become so full

---

[29] The full text of Tennyson's In Memoriam: 45 is located in Appendix A-5.

of itself that it gets too close to the sun. Like Icarus' hubris, narcissism can encourage splendid isolation, a Snow Queen pattern of relating that can condemn to the solitariness of too much distance. *Hiss's* serpentine motions, its physical presence as well as its abstract significance ensure hope's inability to slip out of a dialogue with its opposite. Their reciprocal intimate autonomy promises continued sparks of hope, the sparks negated by no-hope's stings. Now, however, both opposites become tempered with the cooling drops of *hiss*. For the moment, an oppositional dualistic power battle remains structurally thwarted.

The *hiss* of hope adeptly adjusts opposites and invites to a dance of accommodation. The heavens and the earth, life and death begin to move in rhythmic shimmers of light. I am still and I listen to the wise words of the poet: "For what is it to die but to stand naked in the wind and to melt into the sun?" (Gibran, 1932).[30] I try to unleash my ego.

---

[30] The full text of Gibran's poem "On Death" is located in Appendix A-6.

Part Two

Summaries

"Thinking is the art to allow the matter that we are dealing with to speak for itself. ... Thought goes *into* the paradox which *ipso facto* reveals itself as a dialectical contradiction and unfolds its dialectic" (Giegerich, pp. 14-16).

Like the dragonfly, this book unfolds and reveals itself slowly. We remain on the top of the waves of this voyage before we dive in and allow the matter we are dealing with to speak for itself. It "unfolds its own dialectic" but does so gradually, until more and more of the inside becomes the outside. First, there are misty condensations proclaiming the launching of the voyage: the *Summaries*. And then the recording of the actual journey, the transmutations, the molts, testify to the unfolding.

Now

A short summary of present moments of glee, gratitude, and wonder precede the actual Prologue. I have called this short narrative "Now." Symptoms of Parkinson's disease—such as for the most part not being able to walk and being held captive for 5 to 15 hours a day in statue-like immobility; not being able to travel, not being able to give lectures—all these and others seem to have melted (integration?) (Gibran, 1932).[31] After 20 years of Parkinson's violent interruption of my life, I live now more deeply and more bountifully with Parkinson's disease in an intimate autonomy.

"Now" and "Prologue" precede the 16 chapters (small portholes to look out from before the voyage actually begins). Following these short subjective glances, the narrative unfolds from within. Outside manifestations of transmutational moments become evident. The 16 molts, "The Emergence into the Adult Phase," and the "Epilogue" conclude the narrative. Along with the summaries, the chapters, and each molt, these four sections warrant individual attention. I offer a quick glimpse at each.

I have included this narrative device to clarify the networking structures of the book as well as to mirror an experience of *thoughts thinking*—and then going *into* the paradox of an intimate autonomy, often allowing it to *unfold its own dialectic* at its own pace. A *non-egoic* process.

This book is a chronicle of uncovering a viable blueprint for relationship. Gently hovering around the core relationships with Anna and with my husband, the trajectories of the transmutations of relating patterns with the dragonfly and with Parkinson's disease, *The Hiss of Hope* designs and defines the structure of an intimate autonomy. With an interfacing mirror between us all, I find myself often tracing Gibran's developmental dance steps.[32] I feel the energy of—and I observe—our networking plaiting us all together. In and out and out and in—like intricately intertwined notes of music.

Two years after this book ends, Parkinson's disease is still with me. But our relationship has transmuted into one that leaves me with little reason to complain: I am relatively free from movement disorders, I do not fight Parkinson's, nor do I flee from this disease. I do sometimes still

---

[31] "For what is it to die but to stand naked in the wind and melt into the sun." Refer to Appendix A-6 for full text of poem.

[32] The full text of "On Death" is located in Appendix A-6.

freeze going through elevator doors. For the most part, however, I fall; that is, my ego relinquishes agency, and we settle into an intimate autonomy. And embedded in this relating pattern, both Parkinson's and I hover, and we burrow in a tenuously nourishing equanimity.

Prologue

In the beginning there is a flutter. And the flutter gradually surges and vibrates until I seek a source. My body trembles when I hear "Parkinson's disease."

The Prologue introduces "us": Parkinson's disease and me. It also spotlights Anna, my husband, and the dragonfly; we are four partners on this voyage to an intimate autonomous relating pattern. The word *pattern* alludes to the emphasis on structure, on the syntactical facets of an intimate autonomy.

The Hiss of Hope is a walk, a preamble, a proem, through the years 1997 to 2015. But words are used instead of legs or arias. The words weave the beginning of my relationship with Parkinson's disease in and out of the loom of my life. And when a haze of light materializes around me and engulfs my physical form, the word rather shyly and subtly suggests my newly discovered affinity with illness and with death.

From Santa Fe to Frankfurt and now in Edmonton, from a geographical New Mexico landscape of Earth's skin wrapping itself around the Sangre de Cristo Mountains to the financial capital of the world, Frankfurt, Parkinson's and I gradually get to know each other. And now we are in Edmonton, a prairie town in Canada, where not the European waltz but the square dance is in.

We have perhaps always been together, but only since 1997 has he come out of the closet. At first, we do not know how to be with each other. I am told to fight Parkinson's. Or I am told to ignore it, to flee from this disease.

Gradually, slowly, embarking on a voyage through labyrinths of shifting waters, Parkinson's and I encounter difficulties, both in and out of the waves. The challenge is to tread water and to consciously be mindful…an invitation both sparking wonder and igniting terror.

We ultimately find ourselves in an intimately autonomous relationship, in a new pattern of relating.

And all this, a net of words, attending to a narrative that renders me equally to being a not-me; that is, I become my self who is simultaneously not me. Words trace the gradual structural formation of a new space embracing an untried relating pattern, a dynamic dialectical connection between twos. In this space a liquid bridge is spun that enables both a chronic disease and me to shift shapes and mold new configurations of kinetic—and mindful—connections. Words chronicle the transmutation of clashing oppositional constructs to dynamic flowing spaces, of an entanglement in Parkinson's disease, a one, an identification, an "I am Parkinson's" and the transformation to a relationship with Parkinson's, a relating pattern of conversing twos, a self-generating dialectical process, a foundational structure, a blueprint applicable to relationships in general.

Splashed with the waters of a voyage, often transported by the winds generated by dragonfly wings, the me and not-me, my-self and not-self bow our heads to Parkinson's and we all become one. While we are also two. And many.

To employ the word, our mediator, our chosen narrator, most efficiently, I step back and attempt to let it write. However, if moved by the wind or shaken by a thought's thinking, I will pause and succinctly record sudden splashes of compelling insights.

The molts (Latin: *mutare*, "to change")

"Formation, Transformation,
The Eternal Mind's Eternal Animation"
(Goethe, Ed. Trunz, 1986/1996).[33]

---

[33] Gestaltung, Umgestaltung,/Des ewigen Sinnes ewigen Unterhaltung, Faust, lines 6287, 6288.

In Part Two, instead of the word *chapter,* I borrow from the world of biology and have chosen the word *molt.* Molting involves the shedding of an external layer. Molting is about change; it is about reshaping, it is about formation, transformation. Reorganization is the hub of the book.

The book's scaffold of words reflects the planks and the rods, for example, of an architect's sketched designs for the protective and containing structures anticipating the construction of a house. The molts are the forming and the shedding of such structures. The dragonfly, my spirit animal, discards an exoskeleton to expose the naked beginning of a new phase of development, an increased autonomy. For me, each shedding or reconfiguration of a repetition compulsion or of a defense mechanism kindles a new spark of autonomy. I shed an ancient repetitive structure or pattern that for years has held me together and at the same time has held me imprisoned. Due to the increase in the ability to be vulnerable, I experience an increase of autonomy; these moments can provoke an opening to a deepened intimacy, intrapsychically as well as inter-personally. In the case of the house, the scaffold is torn down when the house can stand on its own. For the first time, the house becomes completely visible. The windows can see out as well as in. There is an internal dialectic of light. Without discarding the exoskeleton, the dragonfly's reshaping and formation and transformation are arrested.

Each progression—or regression—is referred to as a molt, a mutation, a transformation. The outer scaffold, the exoskeleton or the inner repetition compulsive structure "dissolves in its own water," and there are space and synaptic sparks for reorganization (Edinger, 1985, pp.76-81).[34] A change becomes inevitable in the structural pattern of networking, of relating.

---

[34] Dissolves in its own water is an alchemical term, part of the process of solutio: "A varient of solutio is liquefactio…dissolved and melted down in order to be recast in new life-forms." For me, this alchemical term is a path to creativity. Without the dissolving, letting go of the need to control, releasing the ego, there is little possibility of allowing the space of creativity to open.

The molts exhibit for the dragonfly, and for me, similar patterns of transmutation. The basic body plans remain the same for both until the emergence of the adult. Then the dragonfly unfolds its wings and flies. I unfold from within and I begin to know new subtle differences, a foreign kind of relationship with the world and with myself. The dragonfly transforms from an immature water-bound insect, or nymph or larva, to an autonomous aerial adult libelle. My transmutation is not such an evident outer change. Rather, it concerns a pattern of relating. Gradually, I learn to know consciously the structure of a more mature intrapsychic and interpersonal connection. I become a participant in new patterns of intimate autonomous relationships.

A new closeness and a new distance become observable between Anna and me, and, reflectively, a new autonomy and intimacy between Parkinson's disease and me. And between me and *me*. Physically and psychically experienced, I can observe the rigid ons and offs of Parkinson's, melting and liquefying into flowing backs and forths and forth and back. Rarely do I now experience being stuck in the opposites. My pattern has more of an ovoid structural form of development, a trajectory encompassing intermittent regressive phases, while the dragonfly's—and the house's—form is more progressive and linear.

When the dragonfly sheds the last exoskeleton, the molting is complete, and the emergence of the adult dragonfly is easy to observe. The previous molts have been obtuse. Therefore, the observing scientist always begins the counting with the adult and calculates backwards. For instance, a larva that molts three times before the final molt to adult was captured at the F-3 stage. No matter how many molts a larva of any species makes, there is no difficulty in determining which one is the last. Reflective of this scientific observational method and mirroring the reorganizational development due to a shedding, a negation, para-doxically employed to further maturation, I designate the first chapter, the first molt, as the last one, consequently placing the last molt as the first. Following the final molt, the dragonfly emerges. The adult phase concludes the formations and transformations.

Words carry and contain the transmuting molts; they generate chaos and turbulence during the voyage and ultimately render their functionality peripheral when the metamorphoses of the dragonfly are complete and promise a free-flying adult. The insect's maturity reflects the human evolution to a free-subsisting adult, a functioning individual who is able to be intimate and vulnerable and therefore autonomous, *I-Moment* assertive, and at the same time able to release ego-structures and fall into a space without structures, without protection of any sort, into a space of nothingness. Here I must learn to play and to dance with the other (Davies, 1928, pp. 55, 113).[35] In a space beyond the word.

A short synopsis of each of the molts offers a preview and an overview of *The Hiss of Hope,* like drops of water witnessing the voyage's unfolding.

Molt 16: Intimate autonomy's anatomy

This molt concentrates on the concept of intimate autonomy, the structural relating pattern integral to this book. The anatomy of this system traces the structures, the constituent configurations of partners in this dialectical paradox. In a relationship harboring this pattern, the twos are not too close, entangled, nor are they too distant, separated. The two glide along the linear skeletal courses into a differentiated one, a unity of diversity, and then back to the two—back and forth and forth and back. And then these opposites melt into each other and form a third, which is a new one. This liquid mercurial dance constitutes the nucleus of the voyage in *The Hiss of Hope*.

Any question or answer concerning the semantics, meaning, or content is irrelevant. We are going to be concerned exclusively with the dynamic endemic to the structure and abstract notion of the anatomy of this relating pattern.

---

[35] Refer to Appendix A-4 for full text of poem "The Dragonfly."

In Molt 16, by way of illustration, I draw from such disciplines as music, poetry, and fairy tales to offer examples that elucidate the structural relating pattern of an intimate autonomy.

And, of course, I draw from my personal experience with Parkinson's disease. Our relating pattern, a fight/flight dualistic structure gradually transmutes into an intimate autonomy. This defensive trajectory of a fight/flight dualism is difficult to bend and then eventually to break. The structure is that of a repetition compulsion and as such has the quality of an indispensable scaffold.

Were I not to emphasize a particular focal point on this voyage in this molt, I would ignore one of the most contemporary notions embedded in Jungian psychology: that of the cultural complex (Singer & Kimbles, 2004). This significant player in North American cultural history is the shamanic spirit animal. For me, it is the dragonfly. Its role is to act as a guide or protector. Although belief in spirit animals—or experience—is indigenous to the First Nations people of North America particularly, it is iconic in belief systems of other cultures throughout history (Oenning-Hodgson, 2009).[36]

Molt 15: "Formation, Transformation,/The Eternal Mind's Eternal Animation"

(*Faust*, lines 6287-6288).[37]

These lines from Johann Wolfgang von Goethe's drama *Faust* are the semantical leitmotifs, as well as the syntactical undertow of Herman Melville's, Goethe's, Anna's, and my—and for that matter, also the dragonfly's—transforming trajectories.[38]

Melville's *Moby Dick* accompanies us on our voyage as a tenuous, white, silvery hoarfrost that crystallizes, reflects, and reveals hidden

---

[36] See my article "Illness as an Illusion of Misfortune" to read more about my "acquisition" of the dragonfly—or his of me.

[37] "Gestaltung, Umgestaltung,/ Des ewigen Sinnes ewige Unterhaltung."

[38] Anna is my central partner in the anaclitic therapy on the voyage into an intimate autonomy.

depths when contrasted with other structures and patterns of relating. These oppositional contrasts illuminate the necessity of carefully calibrating intimacy, as well as distance and autonomy in relationships, while Melville's recognition of Goethe as a kindred spirit emphasizes a surprising synchronicity in the historical, philosophical, and cultural network (Melville, 1847/1967, p. 560).

Molt 14: Anna

Molt 14 introduces Anna. Our analysis in Frankfurt is addressed as well as the subsequent work over the telephone following my move to Edmonton. During the years of minimal contact, Anna's transmutation to a baby whisperer, as well as her honing of the skills of a psychiatric nurse, are traced. Anna's and my decision to enter into an anaclitic therapy is elucidated. Interactions within the guidelines of an anaclitic therapy become the emanating hub of *The Hiss of Hope*. These relating structures ultimately converge, clash; they disconnect and they coagulate into our desired relating pattern.

Molt 13: Alchemical moments and clinical vignettes of the voyage into an intimate autonomy

Molt 13 is long and serpentine. Words and concepts are introduced, and they design forms for potential transformative moments reorganizing into an intimate autonomy (Edinger, 1985, Vol. 12, pp. 52, 53–54, 82).[39] Included are the Red King and the White Queen, their re-

---

[39] In Anatomy of the Psyche, Edinger writes: "In essence, coagulatio is the process that turns everything into earth...heavy and permanent, of fixed position and shape.... Coagulation is often equated with creation...." Jung comments: "The king personifies a hypertrophy of the ego which calls for compensation.... His thirst is due to his boundless concupiscence and egotism. But when he drinks he is overwhelmed by the water—that is, by the unconscious."

formation from two separated entities to two-in-a-one. This trans-mutation can be viewed in the sequence of pictures from the *Rosarium Philosophorum*.

Such concepts as anaclitic therapy, alchemy, syzygy, and *coniunctio* are introduced. The contradistinction between the colors red and white as well as their alchemical conjunction is highlighted and circum-ambulated. The alchemical colors black, white, and red radiate throughout the phases of the opus: the *nigredo, albedo,* and *rubedo.*

At this evolutionary stage in the narrative of *The Hiss of Hope*, and of Anna's and my anaclitic therapy, I introduce the notion of a third space: a wilderness, a horizontal and a vertical place where we learn to dance and to play in anticipation of a mirrored experience of the alchemical union, the Greater *Coniunctio*.[40]

Anna and I become more and more conscious of the necessary two-in-one experience as endemic to our desired relationship, to our human fugue, our intimate autonomy. I highlight our pattern of relating in contradistinction with the too-close projective identification between Ahab and the white whale, as well as the too-distant pattern between Parkinson's and me, our static dualistic fight/flight trajectory.

This differentiation can help to illuminate and to define the depth of the immanent pain and the overwhelming sense of annihilation were Parkinson's and I to remain stuck in this disease's intransigent, oppositional ons and offs. Or if either Anna and I—or Parkinson's and I—were to sacrifice individual potential autonomy through unconsciously falling into Ahab's intimate projective identification pattern of relating with the whale.

In another volume, Edinger describes the king as drowning in the fountain of Aphrodite, the life principle: "A stone there is, and yet no stone,/ In it doth nature work alone,/ From it there welleth forth a fount [Venus-Aphrodite] / In which her Sire, the Fixed, is drown'd/:/ His body and life absorbed therein/ Until the soul's restored agen" (pp. 53-54). This process of solutio is one of the most important in the alchemical procedure. The alchemical opus is often described as solution/(dissolutio) and coagulatio.

[40] The Greater Coniunctio differs from the Lesser Coniunctio in regard to autonomy. To achieve the Greater Coniunctio, there must be enough separation between the Two. This degree of separation, and its attending vulnerability, is an essential ingredient of an intimate autonomy.

Dreams, the steady determination and dedication of both Anna and myself to be open to change, our willingness to hover in the nothingness of a relatively egoless space, our desire to at least touch a two-in-one structural relating pattern, our humor, and our knowledge of the psychic forces—all aid us on this voyage. We are able to shed to some extent the repetition compulsive structures that would impede our endeavors to intuit the cusp of a new consciousness, and thus we are able to continue the voyage into an intimate autonomy.

Molt 12: The dynamic dialectic of play—Galatea

The dynamism of play, the impact and potency of attendant interchange, I recognize and treasure in the myth of Galatea. In this 12th molt, Galatea represents moments of my static quality; she is a mirror of Parkinson's off intervals, of my being rendered immobile.[41] Of my intuiting a state of death. Being off is one of the opposite denoting characteristics of a Parkinsonian movement disorder; the other is being on, an experience of life's animation, life's vitality and vigor.

We hear Pygmalion's desperate plea to Aphrodite that he find a partner as dear to him as his statue. We feel the fire of his impassioned relating pattern to this immobile figure of white stone. Soon after this meeting, Galatea sheds her body of immobile snow-white marble and reveals a human form flowing with red and white hues. She moves her body, she glides through space; I hear echoes of whispers of joy. And of love. From the interaction among Aphrodite, Pygmalion, and Galatea we can sense the power and endemic dynamic quality of this dialectic of play.

I wonder if Parkinson's can be shed.

The third space, this theater of play, we can acknowledge as a wilderness where common laws and rules are not applicable. It is

---

[41] Alchemically, Galatea can be representional of the stone, or the lapis, before—and then after—transformative processes. The "stone that is not a stone."

significant also that we know the third space's function, moreover, as the cryptic creative laboratory of the alchemists. The third space is abstract; it is a notion, a conceptual structure. It is constituted from "the interaction between the subjective and the objective of two worlds, (and then) a third arises of which the expanse is generated thanks to the withdrawal imposed by difference." (Irigaray, 2002, p. 9) This relatively unknown space is essential in its viable pulsating environmental movement, inviting play, communication, and micro- and macrocosmic flowing trajectories of living dialectics. It is also the notion of the Hegelian synthesis, of his thesis/antithesis dialectical dynamic. This notion is the abstract word-form encapsulating our third space (autopoietic self-birthing) that arises thanks to the withdrawal imposed by differences.

Molt 11: The transmutation of the ice mirror

In this molt, I am stuck in a place of paradox and of contradiction, a space of divergent, incompatible notions solidifying into physical experiences of immobility rather than progressing into a third space inviting dynamics of play.

And then suddenly, without any forewarning or hint of imminent change, I can move! I am able to glide independently and freely from one opposite to the other. My body becomes for the first time a guide and an anchor through the labyrinths of the clear opposites of Parkinson's ons and offs as well as through the mists of irrational paradoxical moments in the third space.

As of now, there is no felt connection to the dragonfly except as a conceptual spirit animal.

Molt 10: The dis-union

For the first time, dissension and discord are introduced into Anna's and my collaboration. Perhaps this dynamic is the necessary fire endemic to an optimal oppositional friction igniting "formation transformation,/ The Eternal mind's Eternal animation."

Narcissistically despondent and feeling an inundating aloneness, I collaborate negatively with a white cat from a dream and help her to entangle me defensively once again in my old repetition compulsion of ego-control.

Ego control: An avoidance of vulnerability, an impediment to autonomy. And to intimacy. To closeness. The relationship with Anna is so good, too good. Pulsating with harmony, fun, and mirrored encounters, my psyche shivers with the memory of the physical closeness in the womb and my mother's betrayal after birth. Devoid of conscious awareness, this memory has become a repetitive structure, a mathematical formula: Closeness evokes unthinkable anxiety and pain. To avoid, to hide from such suffering, unconsciously, caught in the impregnable structure of this repetition compulsion, I seek a separation from Anna. This is not a progressive step, but rather it is a regressive defensive move. I do not feel the difference. I am not conscious of the difference. What is not felt or thought remains unchanged and goes further and further inward, deeper and deeper into the well.

Desperately, I feel the need to protect myself. I set up a dualistic relating pattern between Anna and me of right or wrong. Within this dualism, the web of our dialectic and dynamic closeness and independence, our desired relating pattern, is sacrificed. Any consciousness and openness to the alchemical two-in-one union of the Red King and the White Queen seems to have evaporated into a mist of denial. The gliding, sliding, and playing of an intimate autonomy are forfeited.

Upon leaving the third space, I break the protective shell of our balanced relating pattern. I hear the dragonfly's egg crack. While the dragonfly sheds an exoskeleton and progresses, I regress into an aloneness rather than into an autonomy.

Molt 9: The Dragonfly

In this ninth molt, I attach to my spirit animal, the dragonfly, and bow to its guidance. Such moments are not planned; they just happen and seem to settle into a pattern. There is no conscious strategy, nor anticipatory preparation.

I begin to see through the many-faceted eyes of the dragonfly. From a dream, a blind kitten (a metaphorical representative of the mythological blind seer, Tiresias?) collaborates with us. Both the blind eyes of the kitten and the unseeing eyes of Tiresias view through different lenses. I yield to the mastery and guidance of such instances, forces other than my physical body, thoughts of my mind, or matters of will and self-determination. The ninth scaffold (or exoskeleton, or repetition compulsion) is shed. I progress.

Molt 8: The pitbull and the kitten—a two-in-one Movement

A dream ushers two fundamentally different entities together: a pitbull and the normal, adapted kitten from an earlier dream. How can a pitbull and a kitten be a one? The question is raised once again: How can a two be a one at the same time? Is paradox truth? Is a two in one a soul-depth? A two in one implies movement: "the soul is *energeia* (en-erg-eia), the need to express itself and give itself an objective presence ... we could say that the soul is actuosity from the Latin *actuosus*, a rare word meaning full of movement, abounding in action" (Giegerich, 2012, pp. 45-46). For me, a third space is a constituent of this movement.

Molt 7: The egg

The saga of the pitbull and the kitten continues. Once again, I tackle the matter of opposites, a topic endemic to paradox. Opposites can split from each other, remain static, or opposites can encounter each other and enter into a dynamic dialectic. Reflective of my own defensive vertical split, a third space where the pitbull and the kitten could at the least touch each other disappears. A vertical split renders any two dissociative. For a one, the two are too far apart for interaction or interactive dialectics.[42]

With my intrapsychic repetition compulsion pulsating frantically, this clinical split eclipses any trace of a dynamic third space. A split seeks to protect from the probable tension of good and bad oppositional energies. Little room is left for my normal sweet kitten and the raging pitbull to encounter each other and profit from optimal energy derived from clashing friction. They remain as entrenched in their distance as the entangled Ahab and the whale linger, stuck in their closeness. The *hiss* of hope resounds in my ears. My heart beats a bereft counterpoint rhythm.

My ego splits vertically into my old, used, and familiar Snow Queen identification: frozen, always right instead of wrong, and very far away from the soul-truth of paradox. It takes me a long time before I can shed this seventh exoskeleton.

Molt 6: Optimal oppositional friction

I like the rubrical "optimal oppositional friction." I feel another shift in consciousness. I suddenly grasp that I am the pitbull and also the kitten. Both are in my dreams. I am both of them. I am a two in one. And also, I am just me. Parts and a whole (Botoft, 1996).[43] Optimally!

The split eventually yields to a daring dance of syntax and structure, a dynamic movement in a third space. Instead of the split's

---

[42] See Figure 2-A and Figure 2-B, which depict the vertical and horizontal splits in Molt 2. Otto Kernberg and Heinz Kohut concerned themselves with the differentiation between these defense mechanisms in the Seventies. Kohut's contrast of vertical and horizontal splits (1971, p. 193) is almost identical to Kernberg's contrast in splitting and repression. Both see splitting (Kohut's vertical split) as characteristic of a more serious pathology, and repression (Kohut's horizontal split) as a later, less pathological phenomenon.

43 "The everyday awareness is occupied with things (parts). The whole is absent to this awareness because it is not a thing among things. To everyday awareness, the whole is a no-thing, and since this awareness is an awareness of something, no-thing is nothing. The whole which is no-thing is taken as mere nothing, in which case it vanishes. When this loss happens, we are left with a world of things (parts), and the apparent task of putting them together to make a whole. Such an effort disregards the authentic whole."

voracious emptiness, a yawning vacuum riddled with anxiety, the stuck opposites begin to slowly touch each other, and a timid dialogue begins. A networking. How I get there, I still don't know. It is not only about attuned opposition, but rather also about optimal oppositional friction. It's about a partial healing of a split, about the two sides becoming dynamic, entering into a dialectic with each other, playing with each other until eventually they enter into an intimately auto-nomous relating pattern and become a two in one. And a one in two. They become a process self-birthing a new consciousness.

As an example of such a dialectic encounter, I introduce in this sixth molt Jung's notion of active imagination, his conscious drop into the unconscious from 1913-16 after his painful break with Freud. In the recently published *Red Book*, you can find his dialogues with the unconscious as well as his paintings, images of his words (Jung, 2012).

Molt 5: The dragonfly nymph

Molt 5 highlights a structural change. "Formation, Transformation...." While my brain continues to maintain its hegemony over my body, I sense a faint flutter of dragonfly wings and suddenly my body seems to be carried off by the intoxicatingly joyful wind of autonomy. A structural repetition compulsion is shed? At this moment my body rather than my brain sends me messages. And for some unknown reason, this is also the time when I interiorize the dragonfly. Or the dragonfly decides to become a part of me. Or...

The plasticity of the brain is a common contemporary topic of interest. Perhaps neuronal changes can really occur, and Parkinson's can dissolve itself in its own water. Indeed, the parts of my brain exercising control over Parkinson's could morph...or another part of the brain could assume leadership, or perhaps. ... With the shedding of the fifth exoskeleton, I am pregnant with all of this!

Molt 4: The pregnancy

In the fourth molt, I return to questions raised at the end of Molt 5: The first two questions deal with the process of clinical introjection and with the split already referred to in previous molts. The last questions pertain to anaclitic therapy and the world of whiteness. For Anna and for me, the color kindles curiosity and emits whispers of encouragement. We wonder if anaclitic therapy emanates a tinge of whiteness.

The 17th century alchemist Artephius reminds us: "It is the whiteness which quickenth"; Melville describes the terror and the awe Ahab felt while pursuing the white whale.[44] In chapter 42, "The Whiteness of the Whale," Melville depicts the compulsive magnetism of the whale for Ahab. The color is itself replete with sparks of oppositional encounters. The 19th century author explains that, while "whiteness enhances beauty," at the same time it was "the whiteness of the whale that above all appalled" Ahab and fomented Melville's famous question concluding the chapter: "Wonder ye then at the fiery hunt?' (Melville, *Moby Dick*, pp. 163, 170). In the color white all colors are present; their relating demands an intimately autonomous flow; the clash of oppositional moments quickens and can bring forth a consciousness of spaces as yet unknown.

Molt 3: The birth

I feel a skin for the first time in my life: my own living protective structure. External. And correspondingly, the invisible inside turned inside out reveals its hidden function as inwardly protective. Like the ice-mirror: a reflecting exchangeable double-sided part of a whole.

I do not shed my skin, nor does it abandon me. Inside, at the center of my being there seem to be amalgamated deposits of the opposites that once were at war with one another or were stuck in static

---

[44] The Lives of Alchemystical Philosophers, Francis Barrett London, Lackington, Allen & Co. 1815.

opposition. Perhaps their play and dances have gathered together a cluster of energies to form this centrifugal skin as well as a reflective centripetal throbbing center.

Anna's baby-whispering accompaniment as well as the faithfulness to her own center, to her own autonomy, contributes significantly to this process, to this birth.

Molt 2: The split

This second molt finds me spinning the clinical, the scientific, the poetic, and the imaginary together into a web of defensive vertical splits. Once again, a regression to entangled and/or frozen opposites demands a large space in this molt. The scaffolding containment of my repetition compulsion remains defensively protective. My new skin feels tough and taut. There is no shedding possible. In addition, tales of the dragonfly, the balance fly's birthing process, "in a living flash of light he flew," are an important part of this molt, as is Isaac Newton's network of alchemy and gravity.

Molt 1: Anaclitic therapy

In this molt, I return to the foundational stratum of anaclitic therapy. The relating pattern between Anna and me is one of the pivotal keys to my knowing and living an intimate autonomy.

After finally integrating—or dissolving and metabolizing—a key protective repetition compulsive structure, I begin to note and to describe different doors to conscious regression, spaces of relative egolessness, third spaces where one can play and dance. And allow creativity.

In an open exchange, Anna and I talk about our respective experiences, our thoughts and ideas regarding our exposures to anaclitic therapy, and our impressions of how its fallout spills into our everyday lives.

In the middle of this first molt, I have a dream, a dream in which I leave a husk behind.

Part Two

Final Molt: The dance of colors

This is the stage before the emergence of the adult. Once again, it is relevant to emphasize the contrast between the entangled relating pattern of Ahab and the white whale and ours of an intimate autonomy.

In this final molt, I describe how Ahab and the whale sink—perhaps as one or as two—into the blackness of oceanic depths, while the dragonfly sheds its final exoskeleton and flies into a space vibrating with the dynamic of the intimately autonomous relating pattern of a rainbow, an arch of colors mirroring a play space between the heavens and the earth. The white dragonfly's new veneer of many colors confirms its emergence as an adult. And its winged participation in the "internal dialectic of light."

We became aware that the soul is the—uroboric—unity and difference of (a) its own truths and (b) its own potential to perceive, appreciate, reflect and enact those truths, a unity and a difference, moreover, that in Neoplatonic thinking has been expressed in the image of the correspondence of eye and sun, of seeing and shining, we could say: as the internal dialectic of *light*. (Giegerich, 2012, p. 257)[45]

Although the dragonfly has outlived the dinosaur, and there is no question about its capacity to adapt and to undergo metamorphoses, the transmutation of the aquatic larva to the aerial adult is still a wonder of biology. And my emergence to the adult?

****

---

[45] Some say as Two; that is, that Moby Dick lives on. Yet, either way, Giegerich writes, the Two remain in a "unity and difference ... an inner dialectic expressed in the image of the correspondence of eye and sun, of seeing and shining, we could say: as an inner dialectic of light."

The emergence into the adult phase

The head of an adult dragonfly is covered almost entirely by the compound eyes. The optical units that make up these eyes are points of focus that are created by the size, shape, and orientation of these pseudopupils. The dragonfly sees with all of them simultaneously, yet all function together as one unit. A composite image is formed that provides excellent visual discernment. These eyes see rearward as well as forward, and their images burst with color. All this facilitates its ability to detect delectable prey and to elude another predator's greed.

I emerge into my adult phase with the same eyes as before, yet different. How can this be? There seem to be drops of ectoplasm, a viscous substance that is part of the cell that lies just beneath the outer membrane. It is a mysterious entity of liquidity and solidity, a quality of paradoxical presence that ignores the borders of time and space. A spirit entity? A spirit-animal's gift?

In my body, my mind, my way of being, there is a sudden twist, something is different. A paradigm shift? Such a transit is not gradual. Rather, the actual move occurs unexpectedly. Is this mysterious ectoplasmic eye-entity a kind of paradigmatically structured mirror? A sculpted double-sided mirror, an alive eye that reflects and turns and twists, an eye that zeroes in on objects while simultaneously inspecting its own reflected image in its own mirror? I have a giant eye that looks back at itself!

Weird! And yet so simple.

But it is not. Is my emergence into the adult phase due to the eye? Or is the eye mirror a byproduct of the emergence? Or is it an eye dance, a physical movement to prove to myself that I am alive?

Just as a small bird is shoved out of the nest, I, too, feel alone, strange, and quite lost at first. A shedding that breaks open a protective shell in order to emerge is ipso facto terrifying while also exciting because it feeds curiosity and wonder. For me, however, two incidents occur that contribute to an overabundance of dread: Anna becomes so ill that she is hospitalized; John exclaims that he suddenly feels that the role as caregiver has become too much for him. Early memories of helplessness seem to claim my body, my mind, and I endure once again these familiar experiences of being abandoned and disoriented. And anxious.

But then the eye dance begins! An "internal dialectic of light"? The back of my eye sees me. And I see myself reflected as a quantitatively perceived being, in time and space, yet both solid and liquid, both body and mind, both red and white. I am not a nothingness! And I am a nothingness! But I do not have to see myself reflected in my mother's eyes so that I can enter the world as a loved being, as the brilliant Freudian analyst Heinz Kohut postulates (Lachmann, 2008, pp. 7-8).[46] Now I confirm my own existence. I choreograph my own dance! Intimately and autonomously!

I now recognize the adequate distance and I relish the necessarily appropriate intimacy with myself. My sudden emergence into this adult phase...I have no word for this long and difficult process from a place of dissociated helplessness to spaces of intimate autonomous dances. Perhaps there is no word yet. Perhaps there is merely a flash of light announcing the beginning of the end of yet another journey, a journey home, a journey to an intimate autonomy with myself. There must be one word for this mercurial kaleidoscope of sundry moments and diverse data that tenderly flow into a single unity of wonder. Or perhaps two!

Epilogue

Whether it be the center of a storm, a center cut of meat, the center of a flower, or the mirror of the soul, the word that is used to convey this pivotal core is *eye. I? Myself.* Is this center a one of many, a composite of hope and of *hisses*?

---

[46] Heinz Kohut's sparkle in the mother's eyes when she looks at her baby (Glanz im Auge der Mutter) quoted in: Lachmann. See pages 7-9 regarding the difference between "object relations" and "object love."

In "Epilogue," I recall the 28,000 units of the dragonfly's eyes. The central interest of its brain is to collect all the tiny images, to devote 80 percent of this brain to the analysis of visual information, to ultimately observe a picture take form.

Upon being told that I have "ripe" cataracts (and knowing that raspberries cannot be picked until they are dead ripe), I first react with disdain and denial-humor and remark: "I'll wait until they are dead ripe." Above and beyond the fact that the ophthalmologist looked at me as if I were crazy, I felt a terror in the pit of my stomach. An eye operation? It is claimed that the eye and the soul live an intimate autonomy with each other. Is my soul going to be cut off the way Pan is in *The Golden Compass* (Pullman, 1995) [47] ?

Does a cataract operation then effect a paradigmatic shift, a sudden new way of looking at the world? And for myself? Will I then sin no more? Will I—like the dragonfly (both of us adults)—detect "prey and elude greed"? Now that I know that I am no longer a nothingness, now that I am an adult and can see myself as well as the other, now that I can see myself seeing, am I going to have to lose all these new landscapes when the cataracts are exorcised? Is my soul, is the light, going to be forfeited?

Is the centripetal core, the byproduct of years of work in our anaclitic therapy, going to be confiscated? Is everything going to be eviscerated because my eyes do not see as before? I am confident that less than 80 percent of my brain is concerned with my eyes. Or is it? The brain is an *instrument* of the mind. The mind *looks* at things…perhaps the mind is part of the ectoplasm of the eye…

---

[47] In Philip Pullman's The Golden Compass, the Church is convinced that were a child to mature without first being separated from his daemon, or soul, danger becomes inevitable. The Church does not hate children. It fears the inherent potential for sin. The older one becomes, the more conscious one is. And according to Church doctrine, the more aware one is, the more likely he will exercise free will and thus sin. For Lyra, the protagonist of the book, who dearly loves her daemon, Pan, this Church practice seems cruel and dangerous. She feels that she must prove that age or maturity gives her the right to become more aware, that it is the right of all conscious human beings to be able to "sin" —if the Church wants to so name it—and that "to sin" is something necessary and important in life.

But then again...Parkinson's is a brain disease. Perhaps an eye operation changes Parkinson's. And with all the new ideas regarding the plasticity of the brain, perhaps the eye—as a center strand of my personal network—can alter the structure of the brain and thus transmute Parkinson's from a movement disorder to a Galatea-like moving marble. The *dis* of the Parkinsonian's off phase dissolves. The world of sin or no-sin breaks into chaos, into appearances of disorder, into indecipherable data.

There is, however, "no chaos in the universe; the appearance of disorder is merely a function of the limits of perception" (Hawkins, 1995, pp. 42, 138). It is all part of the web, of the network, of life. The eyes of the dragonfly see the myriad points of focus yet view them all simultaneously and know that they all function together as one unit. The off phase of Parkinson's disease moves the dualistic boomerang from the off to the on, and vice versa is transmuted to a circular flow of dragonfly dances with the wind.

Can a dragonfly get Parkinson's? Its brain and its eyes are intimately autonomous. Its brain is an instrument of its eyes...80 percent!

The epilogue describes the cataract operations. Both eyes see differently now. And they are themselves seen. From the back of my eyes, I now perceive the world. And from the front.

Is this the end of the voyage, or is it the beginning? Or am I whirling around in a circle? Past, present, future...hope...*hiss*...what remains loud and clear is not a word, but the sound of *hiss's s: sssssss*... And its echo. And the symmetrical beat of my heart.

Part Three

Transmogrification

Thinking cannot rest content with and stop short at 'paradoxes', 'mysteries', 'the unspeakable', etc. All these terms betray a standpoint that remains outside and perceives from outside. Instead of entering, it stargazes and marvels. Thought goes *into* the 'paradox,' which *ipso facto* reveals itself as a dialectical contradiction and unfolds its dialectic. (Giegerich, 2010, p. 15 fn 21)[48]

Molt 16: Intimate autonomy's anatomy

Intimate autonomy's anatomy is a relating pattern of two—or more— seeking an attunement of dissonant energies and interests into an intimate autonomy—a single—and simultaneously a multifaceted— entity, a one and a many (Jung, 1984, Bd. 14 para 35). This kind of relating pattern can be likened to that of a tree: A tree is a one with many branches. I could imagine each branch searches for the right position to birth itself; it attunes itself centripetally to the oneness of the tree. The more discerning each attuning is, the firmer the tree

---

[48] I have previously brought this quote from Giegerich to the reader's attention. For me, this is one of Giegerich's most important notions.

THE HISS OF HOPE

stands; the more intimately empathetic and vulnerable each branch is to the tree, to its fellow branches, to the sky, and to the snowflakes, the more autonomously and proudly our tree stands. Our tree is rooted securely. It drinks from the nourishing moisture of the earth. Some roots remain gnarled, even bent, and some reach up almost into the heavens when they open themselves and lust for drops of rain.

Another example of an anatomical glimpse into a distant yet simultaneously close relating pattern is illustrated by Bach's "Toccata and Fugue in D Minor"—or any Bach fugue for that matter. But this is my favorite. Listen to the beginning of this piece of music. It is complicated yet simple in its relating pattern of two strands maintaining their respective autonomy while each is simultaneously accommodating and intimately attuning to the notes in the other strand. Gradually, more and more strands are woven contrapuntally into the others already present. Perhaps if we could fall into a fugue, it might be a geometrical pattern that structurally traces our desired relating pattern. And with this interiorization, we could absorb it and know the experience of a many-in-one—and a one-in-many—structure. We can perhaps hear the notes playing and dancing in their paradox of oppositional attunement, while swallowing its anatomy.

A fugue is a fast dance, a dance stemming from the ancient Latin rhythm of *fugere* (to flee) and *fugare* (to chase). The anatomy of an intimate autonomy breaks this dualism. It transmutes an opposition into a dynamically involved dialectic; the one who flees, turns around, and relates to the one who chases. The dancers remain separate, but each contributes to the emergent structure of the polyphonic form, which in turn must reinforce and reflect the individual dancers. At the end of "Toccata and Fugue in D Minor" there is a dying, a moment when every note previously heard dissolves into every note ever heard, and there is an exalted, almost rapturous consummation.

There is another noteworthy and relevant fugue: a poet's fugue of words, which is a poem whose words remain semantically separate. Contrary motion predominates. The words move semantically against each other and create a dissonance. The spaces suspended between

the words, however, allow the syntax to rhythmically catch you. And perhaps rock you in its repetitive pattern. It can feel safe; it can release semantical dissonance and contribute to a feeling of consonance. The dualistic flee and chase yields to an experience—perhaps first of confusion and chaos. There is, however, also a waiting to sense the net's task of weaving disparate parts into a whole, into life's "expression of consciousness in the observable or experiential world of form." (Hawkins, 1995, p. 255) The words' syntaxical dance can also evoke mirthful playing or contribute to a sense, a feeling, of a soothing alignment.

Paul Celan was a Jew who escaped from a concentration camp in Russia after seeing both of his parents executed. For me, one of his most impacting poems is "Death Fugue" (*Todesfugue*). The mere one line startles: "…Death is a Master from Germany" (Celan, 2001).[49]

For our purposes, however, we take yet another line from "Death Fugue" as an example of our verbal anatomical intimate autonomy: "Black milk of daybreak we drink you at night…" These words highlight a paradoxical semantical friction between such words as *black milk* and *daybreak* and *night*. In addition, Celan uses spaces and letters to open up a rhythmic syntax and to allow a structural weaving to lend a contrapuntal dialectic to a piece of poetry. The paradoxical word content, together with the syntactical poetic rhythm, gradually accrue a centripetal center point in spite of the "movement disorder."

Read this poem. It is a fugue and insofar belongs to our Molt 16, but its words semantically concern Germany's failure to live in an intimate autonomy with the Jewish people. The poem encompasses a nation as well as implicating each collaborative individual. It belongs to statements descriptive of a worldwide cultural complex. The words convey warnings about becoming too complacent, too close, or too distant from apparent reality. The structure jars with its placement of words that do not reflect reality, with its disharmonious fugue, a fugue that is not a fugue. It is a poem *about* parts and wholes, and *of* parts

---

[49] The full text of Paul Celan's poem, "Death Fugue" is located in Appendix A-7.

and wholes, about a lens through which both can be seen, about a lens that makes it possible to remain stuck in neither (Bortoft, 1996).[50] It is a death fugue, both semantically and syntactically, both in import and in its structural friction.

The political, historical significance of our individual maturity to know and to practice an intimate autonomy cannot be emphasized too much. Indeed, its failure, or the ignorance of such a pattern of relating, is a historical and contemporary mark of cultural and political shame on us as human beings.

T. S. Eliot is another poet who weaves opposites, or twos into ones. I've already mentioned that in his **"Burnt Norton"** and in *"East Coker"* of *The Four Quartets*, he envisions a "still point," one single serene point, as a requisite for the "dance." And without this still point, there is no dance. This dance is neither still nor in motion; it is seemingly paradoxical. But yet, it "combines the opposites. It mitigates and rectifies all one-sidedness" (Edinger, 1985, p. 215; Eliot, 1943).[51] The more autonomous each opposite is, the more intimate it can be. The defining quality is vulnerability. Openness.

The anatomy of our relating pattern, a physical mirror of a two-in-one relationship, a structural representation of an intimate autonomy can be outlined if we think of an embryo in the womb of the mother. The intimacy of blood and oxygen exchange can only occur if each of the two is autonomous in their intimacy. For the first months after birth, a diagrammatic sketch does not change: These two are still one unit. Psychoanalyst D. W. Winnicott maintains there is no such a thing as a baby: There is only a baby and a mother (Winnicott, 1971, p. 34).

---

[50] Bortoft's book is an excellent book to recommend regarding the scientific way of looking at parts and "seeing" wholeness as well.

[51] The culmination of the alchemical process, the Philosopher's Stone, describes itself: "I am the mediatrix of the elements, making one to agree with another; that which is warm I make cold, and the reverse; that which is dry I make moist, and the reverse; that which is hard, I soften, and the reverse. I am the end and my beloved in the beginning. I am the whole work and all science is hidden in me."

Part II of Jung's *Mysterium Coniunctionis*, "The *Paradoxa*," cites example after example of paradoxical twos being superseded by a new plane on which the difference between positivity and negativity is now categorical and "you need the Dionysian frenzy of dialectical logic to deal with it." (Jung, 1971, Bd. 14/1, pp. 62-113; Giegerich, 1998, p. 148) The conclusion of Goethe's *Faust* exemplifies a play with words, an intimate autonomous word game, a closeness, and then just enough distance to invite the need to closely examine what the words could possibly mean. The reader is seduced into a space of perpetual motion. Each couplet presents a paradox, an incongruity, a contradiction. Each contradiction structurally nudges forward with a semicolon or a comma. There is no period to invite relaxation. The semantical paradox vibrates and forces the reader to move. The structural linguistic tools of punctuation and positioning play with the semantics of the words. The challenge to comprehend meaning or stop and meditate on a particular word is difficult. It feels as if you are syntaxically vibrated onward. Until the period at the very conclusion. The intimate autonomy of the syntax and the semantics, the structural punctuation that separates and does not separate, and the rhyme and the rhythm, the meaning and the nonsense...all play with each other. If one does not go with the flow, if you do not play, it is an empty pastime, or fight and flight enter the dynamic, and frustration remains as residue. These are *Faust*'s concluding words:

> *Everything transient*
> *Is merely a mirror.*
> *The things abstruse*
> *Become soon clear,*
> *The nameless*
> *Here, it is always sung*
> *The eternal feminine lures us on.*
> (Faust, Part 2, Oenning-Hodgson, trans., lines 12104–12111)[52]

---

[52] Alles Vergaengliche/Ist nur ein Gleichnis;/ Das Unzulaengliche, Hier wirds Ereignis;/ Das Unbeschreibliche,/ Hier ist's getan;/ Das Ewig-Weibliche/ Zieht uns hinan.

Indeed, relating in an intimate autonomy implies movement, dynamic dialogue, a space, a third space where oppositional tension dances until even the slightest slender balance initiates a flow of dialectical melodious accommodation. "The two intertwine, in each one and between one another, so as to build a possible dwelling for humans. Time itself becomes space…in a listening to oneself and to the other, and also to that third which arises." (Irigaray, 2002, pp. 148, 149)

The notion of this relating pattern of an intimate autonomy came to me while discussing with a colleague what the goal of an analysis is. Having lived in Germany for so long, I instantly remembered Hans Dieckmann's emphasis on an ego that could carry suffering (*ein leidensfaehiges Ich*). In a lecture at a DGAP (*Deutsche Gesellschaft Analytischer Psychologen* — The German Society of Analytical Psychologists) conference, he had emphatically declared that with such a strong ego one could go through life successfully. I remember thinking that such a concentration on the ego was not enough for me. The next colleague interviewed replied that, for her, the goal of analysis was to be able to hold the intensity of the divine. One man said that, for him, the central emphasis in analysis was to "feel whole." There were more answers, but as Adorno emphatically states: "The positivists are always right, but they seldom speak the truth." In other words, there is no right or wrong. If one is entangled in being right or wrong, the truth can be lost in this dualistic power battle. Indeed, if one is stuck in a dualistic flee and chase, the truth about the goal of analysis gets lost. The truth lies in all of the former and many more.

On our voyage, the important goal is not to get caught in one or the other but to flow back and forth and forth and back. One could say the goal is to learn to live in the fugue of an intimate autonomy. At this moment, for me the most important goal is to know a distance and a closeness endemic in a *we* in the throes of a constitutive dynamic dialectic between ones, twos, etc. Next year, however, it could be something else.

Fairy tale blueprints of an intimate autonomous relating pattern

To elucidate further the notion of an intimate autonomy, there will be clinical examples of these moments in the relationship between Anna and me from our anaclitic therapy. To illuminate this sphinxlike paradoxical relating pattern first, however, in more general terms I can illustrate this relationship structure as viewed from a literary, more collective, cultural context. First, I want to recount two fairy tales: one, in which there is too much autonomy, too much distance; and one in which the intimacy is too close and becomes a golden cage. As in most fairy tales, the protagonists must suffer, solve riddles, and travel great distances to become more conscious. With the newly won *other* in both fairy tales, we can sense a space that can unfold a hidden propensity to an intimate autonomous relating pattern.

In this first fairy tale, there is too much autonomy, too much distance in the relating pattern between the wren and the eagle.

The king of the birds

Once upon a time a meeting was called for all the birds in the kingdom. They were to come together to select a king or a queen, who would function as a centripetal figure, a centering force around which the birds could all gather. With such a movement towards a containing and firm center, their present distress of disconnection suffered throughout the kingdom could be eased. The majority of the birds had complained of feeling aimlessly scattered, alone and even homeless. Single birds did not feel as a part of a whole.

It was proclaimed that a competition would take place, a race to see who could fly the highest. He or she would then be declared the ruler of the kingdom and would become the centering matrix they all yearned for.

Some of the birds chirped among themselves, intimidated because they all assumed that the eagle would join the competition and that she would win. They all knew how strong she was, how powerful, and how arrogant, and they wondered if any of them would have a chance competing against her. And they conjectured that the eagle's attitude would diminish her abilities to harmonize dissonant and consonant elements. Could she become a centripetal energy?

But they all yearned for a center and a firm and defined secure space, where they could all gather and feel as One.

And so the race was declared on.

The day of the race arrived, they all lined up, the start signal was given, and they took off. They flew and they flew, straight up into the Heavens. The eagle did not even look around at first. She knew that most of the smaller birds would give up quickly. But as fewer and fewer were left in the skies, she began to watch. She noted when the last bird still flying gave a sigh, let his tired wings fall, and glided back to earth.

The eagle laughed to herself, spread her beautiful wings, felt her majesty and her power, flew a few exhibitionistic circles in the sky and then turned toward the earth. At that moment, a small wren, who had hidden in the eagle's feathers and had flown snuggled and relaxed on the eagle's back, gave a tiny leap into the Heavens. He was declared the winner and became the King of the Birds, clever, wise, and creative. And he embodied a consolidating force yearned for by all: the strength of vulnerability, the warmth of intimacy, and they all intuited a new relating pattern: an intimate autonomy for each and for all (Grimm & Grimm, 1884/1981).

Our little wren had won. He had perhaps demonstrated what creativity can look like: He had ridden on the back of history, he had carried out an unusual and rather intuitive spark of wisdom, he had demonstrated that the smallest leap into some place totally new can bring a kingdom into existence. But after the excitement wore off, our little wren was alone. And he felt lonesome. "Is this what I wanted?" he asked himself. "Are all kings so alone?" Our little wren looked around and noticed his former partner for the first time. The eagle flew high, she flew long, she flew here and there, but she seemed to be despondent. Her wings appeared limp, her eyes emptied of their one-time flashes of power, of arrogance, of self-confidence. The birds had a center now holding them all together, but there was no dynamically connecting third space of play, of empathy. There was no intimacy.

Too autonomous, too distant, too separated, and too alone, the wren and the eagle and the rest of the birds soon recognized a collective shroud of depression settling down onto each of them, and they felt a need to dialogue. Karen Armstrong writes that, in a true dialogue, each participant must make a place for the other in his mind, listening intently and sympathetically to the ideas of his partner in dialogue and allowing them to unsettle his own convictions. In return, they would permit their minds to be informed and changed by his contribution. (Armstrong, 2011, p. 132)

And so it was. A new centripetal center gradually became firmer and firmer, it became a space of robust intimacy. The spaces between the birds once filled with a cacophony of dissonant melodies became an opera of interfacing arias. And they all—and each—soon knew that with the eagle and the wren together as their sustaining matrix—plus their recently discovered space of play and dialogue, if this new pattern of relating would not be lost, that they could live happily ever after. And if they are not dead yet, they continue to live in their new relating pattern of an intimate autonomy.

The other fairy tale to be told is one of too little distance and too much closeness.

Florinda and Yoringal

Once upon a time, long, long ago, a young maiden, Florinda, and her new husband, Yoringal, were walking in the woods. They were each so intimately involved with the other that any spark of autonomy for either one of them had been sacrificed and lost in the entanglement of being too close. It is no wonder that they both failed to keep track of any sense of direction and soon they found themselves lost in dark, deep woods.

A witch, who lived in the darkest part of the forest, collected beautiful young maidens. She changed them into nightingales, imprisoned each in a golden cage, and hoped that the geographical intimacy of their youth, their beauty, and their music would spill out between the bars and bring a surplus of these qualities into her world. She could then avail herself of them any time she pleased. Of course, she was only interested in herself. Not in a relationship.

The witch caught Florinda and put her in an especially beautiful golden cage. Before she could turn Yoringal into a statue of stone, he took off as fast as he could and he ran and ran and ran. Far, far away in high mountains, he finally stopped.

Seven long and lonely years he spent there as a shepherd. His only company were the white sheep he had gathered around him. And even though he yearned for Florinda, he gradually lost the burning need that had consumed him before. His loneliness transformed into solitariness and reorganized itself into a firm and deep autonomy.

And then it came to pass that he had a dream, a dream so real that he knew to follow its message: He was to search for a flower, a flower with petals as red as blood and with a center as white as snow. Only with this flower in his possession would he know a relating pattern that promised the awareness of a distance and a closeness conducive to a healthy and mature relationship. Only with this flower in his possession could he free Florinda. He found the flower in a crevice on the very top of a mountain. Only when the sun's rays illuminated this strange flower, did it not remain concealed.

Both the red petals and the white center seemed to come alive as he picked it. Holding it in his hand, he perceived a pulsating rhythm like a heartbeat. Despite their differences in color and hue, in texture and in density, despite the oppositional features of this flower—the red and white, the soft yet solid petals and the dewy liquid center—despite these anti-thetical components, the flower radiated a concordance, a chaotic harmony yet unknown to Yoringal. Despite the fact that Yoringal had been separated from Florinda for seven long years, he suddenly felt as before, but yet at the same time, he felt a kind of altered love for her. A more distant love, a more autonomous connection. And more curious than driven, he began the long trek home.

Of course, first he went into the forest and into the witch's house. Yoringal recognized the golden cage of Florinda immediately. He touched the cage with the flower, the bars disintegrated, and Florinda shed her nightingale feathers to become the maiden she once was. And was not. For the long years *without Yoringal had likewise imbued her with wisdom beyond her young years, a wisdom of a more mature and deep relating pattern.*

They must have lost the red flower with the white center on their way out of the forest. The witch happened upon it and knew the flower for what it was: a Promethian secret stolen from the Heavens! A flower of the Earth divulging the cryptic core of love everlasting, a flower bridging opposites, heralding something new: the white of the Heavens and red of the Earth in the fecundity of a cyclical dialogue with each other. And the witch watched over the flower and kept it flourishing in her secret garden. Soon her interest in collecting young maidens began to wane; she began to yearn for a relationship akin to the white and the red of the flower. And it just so happened that when taking a walk in her woods on a sunny afternoon, the witch ran into a brilliant wizard. It was not long before they began to live together in harmony…and in occasional dissonance. The witch knew then that she and the wizard would live happily ever after. And if they are not dead, they are still alive and prosper in their unusual intimate autonomy. (These words are the actual ending of Grimms' fairy tales. The translation into English is: And they all lived happily ever after.) (Grimm & Grimm, 1884/1981, p. 247)

Personal experiences of an intimate autonomy

The structural composition, the anatomy of an intimate autonomy, I can elucidate ad infinitum, and I can use words to further clarify and exemplify. It is also appropriate to describe my own personal participation in this relating pattern. In agreement with Faust when he concluded: "In the Beginning was the deed." (Goethe, 1806/1992, Trans. M. Greenberg, line 1237)[53] I want to be able to *live* this pattern and relate the key moments of such experiences. I don't want to wait seven years for a dream, nor do I want to hope for an enchanted flower.

---

[53] "Im Anfang war die Tat."

Any further diatribe over meaning discourages and digresses from our original intent to record actual configurations of this two-in-one relating pattern experienced on this voyage.

Molt 15: "Formation, Transformation, Eternal Mind's Eternal Animation"

"Form follows function — that has been misunderstood.
Form and function should be one, joined in a spiritual union."
Frank Lloyd Wright (1939)

And all of a sudden, Anna is here, and we begin the voyage. It has been as narrated above, a violent, difficult, and awesome journey into a new exposure of being together and being separate, a space filled with moments of attuned as well as dynamically dissonant opposition. We have flown on the notes of Bach's fugue, we have rested in spaces where we could dance and yet be filled with stillness, spaces where we could breathe together intimately while each celebrates autonomously her "Last Supper" according to Jung's admonition: We must each drink our own blood and eat our own flesh (Vol. 14, para. 512). And—if we are able and willing to transform and recreate—we can hope for the experience of a higher health, while simultaneously listening for hope's inevitable *hiss*.

And with the grace and beauty of the eagle and the humbleness, instinctive wisdom, and creativity of our little wren, with the love of Yoringal and Florinda touching our hearts while the wisdom of the witch and the wizard mirror the twoness of the colors, white and red in one flower, we begin to live and to relate in the pattern of an intimate autonomy. Tarrying with aloneness, a fugue of a multitude of hues, sometimes clashing, often complementary, while dancing with the still melodies and contrapuntal pieces of kaleidoscope glass and mirrors, we learn to recreate pictures that often fall together due to the optimal oppositional friction and fractals of light polarization. And tracing patterns of relating in our own cells while each drinks and digests her own blood, like a magic feast, we suddenly recognize that our individual loneliness sometimes transmutes to solitude, our vulnerability to autonomy. *And if we are not dead yet, we are still living.*

Joining us on this voyage is a motley crew of Germans and Americans. Herman Melville, in a letter dated June 1851, referred to Johann Wolfgang von Goethe's poem, written in 1821, "One and Everything" (*Eins und Alles*): "This 'live in all' feeling…there is some truth to it…lying in the grass on a warm summer's day. Your legs seem to send out shoots into the earth. Your hair feels like leaves upon your head. This is the *all* feeling" (Melville, 1847/1967, p. 560).

That Melville's understanding of the poem as being about a too-close relationship, that is, a relating pattern of participation mystique with nature instead of an intimately autonomous relating pattern, is evidenced in his great novel, *Moby Dick*. Ahab, the captain of the ship, voyages long, he voyages hard, in order to wound the whale, Moby Dick, who has earlier attacked Ahab and left him with but one leg. A wound for a wound! Ahab leaves no space for dialogue—or for a dance—with the white whale, no room for time and space to offer a flower of attuned opposites. Ahab feels a compulsion to reflectively harm that which has harmed him. Not the slightest distance or autonomy does he grant himself or Moby Dick. Ahab views the whale as a projection of himself—his "*all* feeling." They are a one without any trace of Goethe's *Two in One*.

Ultimately, after harpooning the white whale and seeing him bleed black blood, Ahab's line catches around his own neck. The captain of the ship and the whale both disappear into the depths of the mighty ocean. It is left open whether Moby Dick once again is viewed in the midst of stormy waves, or whether the white whale, wounded and alone, dies and is buried in the ocean's depths along with Ahab. A statement of nature confirming Melville's recognition of Goethe's poem? (Melville, 1847/1967, p. 560)

In Ahab and Moby Dick's relating pattern, there is no space for dialogue; there is no space to dance, to play, either together or alone. Nor is there the slightest pulsating potential of Goethe's higher health. For Goethe, health is not freedom from illness and suffering. Instead, it is our task to not get caught in, to not identify with, the opposites of well or not well, but to learn to move to the rhythm of an oppositional attunement between health and sickness, as well as to flow from any one opposite to the other. In his words, higher health is the achievement of this relating pattern. This summit can only be reached through using something like the fine-tuning of an artist toward life itself (*eine Lebenskunst*). Goethe's higher health is the patient's attitude toward illness and his or her ability to let go of old patterns and to be open to change. These famous lines in *Faust* are leitmotifs throughout this great drama:

> I am not me if I stay stuck.
> Awe and fear are man's inalienable luck;
> It doesn't really matter how the world views it,
> I want to know the depth and the dearth of life's worst lot. ...
> Whatever will be, will be. Formation, transformation,
> Eternal Mind's eternal animation.
> (Goethe, *Faust*, Trans. Oenning-Hodgson, lines 6271–6287, 6288)[54]

Molt 14: Anna

In the last five weeks, Anna and I have been conjuring up surging waves of energy. For me, she has been an anchor, a guide, and she has been an Ahab, albeit without Melville's misunderstanding of Goethe's poem "One and Everything" (*"Eins und Alles"*). While involved in this whale-chasing journey, sliding along the undulating crest of an ocean's infinity,

---

[54] Doch im Erstarren such' ich nicht mein Heil,/ Das Schaudern ist der Menschheit bestes Teil;/ Wie auch die Welt ihm das Gefuehl verteure,/Ergriffen, fuehlt er tief das Ungeheure.... Wie es eben kommt. Gestaltung Umgestaltung,/Des ewigen Sinnes ewige Unterhaltung.

yet at the same time sustained, restrained, and contained by time's dearth of eternity, we have been able to extend our search into the hitherto untried horizons of watery depths. Significant elements, such as the third space's playful nondualistic patterns, reflective of Anna's previous analysis with me, we sight and recognize as potentially constructive, signposts for transformational relating to symptoms of early trauma, its usual reactive fight/flight response, as well as to symptoms indicative of a chronic illness. Specifically, to my illness: Parkinson's disease.

In Germany, I practiced as a Jungian psychoanalyst from 1985-99. Professionally, there is a clear differentiation between psychoanalytic work and other forms of therapy. Germany is one of those rare countries where individual health and psychological health are considered to be a collective concern. After we practitioners submit a detailed anamnesis of any given patient to an approved evaluator, the German Federal Ministry of Health (Bundesgesundheits Ministerium) can decide to subsidize three years of analytic work. If substantially defended, the analytic work can be extended. The stipulation is that the patient comes at least twice a week. Otherwise, there is thought to be too much space in between where defenses can be built up again.

According to the regulative issued by the Federal Ministry of Health, the two moments that differentiate analytic work from other therapy forms are *regression* and *transference*. Both the psychic regression and the transference, this outer interpersonal experience (for example, an initial projection of a personal negative mother onto the analyst and its transmutation into a good-enough mother) becomes the inner intrapsychic structure that can eclipse a neurotic repetition compulsion.

Anna began her analysis with me in Frankfurt in 1991, 27 years ago. At that time, she had been advised by a senior Freudian psychoanalyst to enter a mental institution, to give up hope of ever being able to withstand analysis, and to have herself medicated as soon as possible. Today, I know of no one as autonomous and simultaneously as related as Anna. She is firmly rooted in her own center. She explains: "I knew my analytic work had granted me my life back when I recognized my ability to give myself without losing myself."[55]

Anna and I worked together in Frankfurt for eight years. After my move to Canada in 1999, we decided to continue analysis by telephone, one hour a week. She paid for the hours privately. In June of 2001, we terminated our analysis.

I had minimal contact with Anna after that. After some years, Anna called to say that she is visiting a cousin in Victoria and would like to come to Edmonton for a short visit. During this weekend stopover, Anna notes my difficulty with Parkinson's and on the telephone later she exclaims: "I am a nurse and your 'daughter.' It is time that this grateful daughter gives something back to the mother."

An experienced pediatric and psychiatric nurse, at 53 years of age, Anna decides to supplement her income by initiating her own baby-whispering enterprise.[56] After a series of interviews in London, she is listed with international agencies as a maternity nurse seeking employment.

Her first call comes from Munich. A mother of two boys tells Anna that her usual nanny has suddenly canceled and asks if it would be possible for Anna to come right away. Pregnant, this mother explicitly emphasizes the necessity for Anna to focus on getting the newborn on a fixed schedule as quickly as possible. She and her husband are both immersed in their respective professions, as well as having to deal with

---

[55] German translation: "Ich kann mich hingeben, ohne mich aufgeben zu muessen."

[56] Anna borrowed the expression baby whisperer from the term horse whisperer. The success of novels like that of Nicholas Evans (1995)—and the subsequent film—has made horse whisperer a common description referring to the emphasis on kindness, with particular concentration on communicating with—and learning to understand from the horse's point of view—the natural behavior of horses. Equally important is the emphasis on the horse becoming a human whisperer; that the horse become adept at recognizing and following "suggestions" made by the horse whisperer. This culminates in a relating pattern of an intimate autonomy. Not surprisingly, a great many horse owners turn to horse whispering in the belief that these horsemanship methods offer something that will give them a closer, more trusting relationship with their horses. Nor is it surprising that Anna would imagine that the same pattern could be particularly appropriate for relating to infants.

two other children. With an apologetic yet firm tone, Anna explained that she is a baby whisperer and cursorily summarized attachment theory, concentrating on D. W. Winnicott's idea of playing. In addition, Anna explains, for Winnicott there is no such a thing as a baby. "When you set out to describe a baby, you are describing a dyad, baby *and* someone…a baby is ipso facto part of a relationship" (Davis & Wallbridge, 1981, p. 35). If she were willing to come, she would be there for the newborn and for the mother, herself as primary caregiver, as well as for the dyad of the biological mother and the newborn. She would concentrate on the two in one, the one-in-two exchange and flow. She would listen to and she would follow the language of the baby's breath, referred to medically as *air hunger*. Together, she and the newborn determine the trajectory of their relating pattern.

The mother hired Anna on the spot. Anna's reputation as an unusual and exceptional maternity nurse began with her baby-whispering experience in Munich and with this mother's effusive recommendations. The ability to *hear* the newborn, to communicate with the varied whispers of the baby's breath, with the primal feeling tones of words, with the sensate touch of skin, Anna's preverbal interaction with the infant, as well as her inclusive interpersonal interaction with the mother were soon reflected in a spiraling demand from other expectant mothers for her quality of presence.

Anna's and my individual histories, experiences and professions, the shared respect for "whispers," our separate lives along with the recognition of common interests and proclivities, our discovery of a mutual glow after shared humor as well as an enjoyment of mature—and immature—fun, plus a parallel sense of irony, these prevalent attributes plus obvious individual and cultural differences, all have contributed to a mutual decision to enter into our anaclitic therapy. This experience becomes the voyage into the process, into the form and the function, of our desired relating pattern, into an intimate autonomy.

Molt 13: Alchemical moments and clinical vignettes of the voyage into an intimate autonomy

Actaion and Artemis are not *really* two separate and very different (indeed opposite) beings, male versus female, human vs. goddess. Both *together* are the soul, one and the same soul, which here, however, *unfolds* itself into a syzygy of opposites in order to realize itself as the Notion.... The unity *of* unity *and* difference.... (Giegerich, 1998, p. 208)

***

Alchemy is the transformation of consciousness; it is a paradigm shift (such as Nicholas Copernicus must have experienced when he suddenly 'knew' that the earth revolved around the sun, instead of vice versa). Paradox is a key to higher consciousness. To accomplish this great work, however, one must move beyond paradoxical thinking. When the Red King and the White Queen are 'married', the child of light is born. This is alchemical, the transformation of consciousness. (Caris, 1987, p. 173)

For this long and serpentine chapter, terminology worthy of special attention is listed below:

- *Opposites*: diametrically different
- *Paradox*: a self-contradictory statement, from the Greek word *paradoxon* that means contrary to expectations, existing belief, or perceived opinion
- *Alchemy*: the medieval forerunner of chemistry, based on the transformation of matter. "An old alchemical dictum says: 'dissolve the matter in its own water.' This is what we do when we try to understand the process of psychotherapy in terms of alchemy" (Edinger, 1985, p. 1).
- *Syzygy*: a pair of connected or corresponding things. The "two" form a "third."

- *Coniunctio*: "The 'lesser *coniunctio'* is a union or fusion of substances that are not yet thoroughly separated or discriminated. It is always followed by death or *'mortificatio.'* The 'greater *coniunctio,'* on the other hand, is the goal of the opus, the supreme accomplishment." (Edinger, 1985, p. 211)

Alchemical moments

The second time Anna returns to Edmonton, she is here for six weeks.

Ours is a strange relationship. An unusual relationship. A daring voyage.

Reflective of Anna's analysis with me, and being familiar with the clinical matrix of anaclitic therapy, we try to use the force and friction of regression, of a decrease in ego-control or subjective functioning, to agitate an equilibrium.[57] In a space of regression, a chaos, an opening prevails in which reorganization, a reforming of embedded structural patterns is possible. Ultimately, I will be concerned with the sighting and the unraveling of repetition compulsive structures, of memories stored in the body. These configurations can first protect us, then they confine us, indeed they hold us captive. We are destined to remain stuck if these addictive compulsions are not released into a regressive space, tamed, and changed. Hope and no-hope, and *hiss* until all three drown in their own waters. The sibilant gift of *hiss* opens a space of potential, of new dynamic dialectics, of possible transformations.

---

[57] The concept of anaclitic therapy was introduced in 1946 by psychiatrist Rene Spitz to refer to children who became depressed after being separated from their mothers for a period of three months or longer during the second six months of life, since these children had no one to lean on for the nurturance they required. Spitz coined the term anaclitic (from the Greek anaklitos—"for reclining") depression to identify their condition. Anaclitic therapy, a little-known chapter in the history of North American psychoanalysis and psychiatry, sheds light on the prevailing trends and therapeutic approaches common in the 1950s and 1960s. It touches upon major junctions in the history of psychoanalysis and psychiatry such as the therapeutic use of regression, the usage of biological measures in conjunction with psychoanalysis, and the relationship between the therapist and patient. See Molt 1.

Since we are on a voyage, we can picture a regression that causes oceanic waves to become turbulent and to surge into sources of reorganization. We conjecture that in my case a breaking wave, a wave whose base can no longer support its top, causes a collapse, and a crack is then opened through which Parkinson's slips in and captures me. I am swept into either an entangled relating pattern with Parkinson's, a too-close relationship, or I am frozen into separation, a too-distant pattern. In both cases I am off. Parkinson's is likewise off. Entangled, it lives out its rapacious identity; separated, it is compelled to exist alone, disconnected yet connected. For us both, moments of a "unity *of* unity *and* of difference" (Giegerich, 1998, p. 120) dissolve into mists of evanescent memory.

If the wave could connect with its base and thereby close this liquid fracture, Parkinson's and I could discover a nondualistic relating pattern; perhaps we would learn to play with the flowing water of the wave to relate dynamically with each other. And perhaps we can enter into the desired relating pattern of an intimate autonomy. A paradox. Raymond Weaver's comment in 1919 about Melville's *Moby Dick* is good advice when dealing with a paradox: "If one logically analyzes *Moby Dick*, he will be disgusted. ... If one will forget logic and common sense, and abandon himself...to this work of Melville's, he will acknowledge the presence of an amazing masterpiece," (Melville, 1847/196, p. 626, 627)

Our intimate autonomy is a paradox that demands one abandons oneself to the feeling and to the notion of both the intimacy and the autonomy while simultaneously noting the potential flow when both are conceived together. I can be intimately together with Anna, when we discuss, for example, the dragonfly and my attachment to a spirit animal, and at the same time, we are both autonomous with our contradictory opinion. A paradox is relationship, a containing vessel. A circular form is assumed; it is a dynamic, a moving relating structure. A form that can open a new and fresh consciousness, a space beyond the paradox. To a space where dualistic tension dissolves, "where eyes do not have the function to see. Instead, eyes are 'opened' to a new dimension" (Giegerich, 2010, Vol. 4, p. 510, n. 8). To recapitulate: intimacy requires the ability to give of oneself without losing oneself, while autonomy necessitates an openness, a vulnerability. An ability to "stand naked in the wind"—as the poet writes (Gibran, 1932).[58]

The paradox and beyond

One of the major principles of alchemy is the *coalition of opposites.* Opposites are twos. A separation of these twos is the initial nonrelating moment in the alchemical process of the transformation of consciousness. Each one of the two enters into a process of depth psychotherapy; in alchemy this process is an opus. As Edinger writes, it is a sacred work. ... Patience is basic. Courage means a willingness to face anxiety. Continuous regimen means that through all shifts of mood and mental state one is willing to persevere in the effort to scrutinize and understand what is happening. (Edinger, 1985, p. 5)

The more intimate and the more autonomous each one of the two becomes, the more both become dynamically and dialectically involved. Alchemy's unification—or *coniunctio*—is intimate autonomy's trajectory deforming from a straight or elliptical to a circular con-figuration. A form whose beginning and end remains cryptic in its circularity. A form that *feeds energy back to itself* (feedback), a form whose uroboric quality invites a *perpetuum mobile*, a sustained energy, that promises an ultimate spiraling snaky transformation. This energy becomes the object of centrifugal as well as centripetal forces; the relating pattern opens beyond the horizontality of a paradox. It touches the verticality of the eternal and of infinity. Kairos moments. Form claims the position of the subject and of object concommitantly and then can dissolve into itself. A position beyond the paradox where truth and creativity abide.

---

[58] The full text of Gibran's poem On Death is located in Appendix A-6.

The process of a transformation relies on the intimate autonomous relating pattern of Two, like the alchemical marriage of the Red King and the White Queen. Light—or consciousness—is their child.[59]

C. G. Jung corroborates that a separation, an experience of twos, is necessary for further consciousness, but he notes the negation of consciousness were the twos to become too far apart. He writes:

> The tendency to separate the opposites as much as possible and to strive for singleness of meaning is absolutely necessary for clarity of consciousness, since discrimination is of its essence. But when the separation is carried so far that the complementary opposite is lost sight of, and the blackness of the whiteness, the evil of the good, the depth of the heights, and so on, is no longer seen, the result is one-sidedness. (Edinger, 1995, p. 210)

If even one of the separated twos can begin to move, the opposites have the possibility, however, to reform into a paradox. Jung explains that these opposites have the opportunity through their unity and their difference to become a paradox. He emphasizes the preeminent role this *unification* plays for the alchemist and contributes gems of intricate passageways inherent in paradoxical patterns of relating (Jung, 1984, Bd. 14/1, pp. 62-113). And he warns:

> We should not begrudge the alchemists their secret language: deeper insight into the problems of psychic development soon teaches us how much better it is to reserve judgement instead of prematurely announcing to all and sundry what's what. Of course we all have an understandable desire for crystal clarity, but we are apt to forget that in psychic matters we are dealing with processes of experience, that is with transformations which should not be given hard and fast names if their living movement is not to petrify in something static...this is just as important...a re-experiencing of that twilight which we can learn to

---

[59] John Caris, Foundation for a New Consciousess, Chapter 5. Westgate House, 1987.

understand only through inoffensive empathy, but which too much clarity only dispels. (Edinger, 1985, p. 15)

In this space of twilight, the child of light is born.

To illustrate and to illuminate this point of transition, this new cusp of consciousness, I want to unravel the relating patterns of the following opposites, of the twos and their respective journeys to intimate autonomous positions: Parkinson's and I, Anna and I, John and I, the dragonfly and I. The colors red and white carried by the alchemical King and Queen belong also to a transformation provoked by paradoxical energies. The 1550 series of pictures, *Rosarium Philisophorum*, depict their oppositional development from a relating pattern of too much distance to a balanced intimate autonomy, a dance of red and white. Jung has published prints of the famous woodcuts depicting their transformation into an intimate autonomy in his book titled *The Psychology of the Transference*.

"The unity of unity and difference...." (Giegerich, 1998, p. 120)

Parkinson's and I

Clinically, caught in the Parkinson's syndrome, one is catapulted from being on to being off throughout the day and throughout the night with the *hiss* of the gasps in between. This physical experience reflects the more psychological repetition compulsion of the unconsciously egoic reactive, dualistic fight/flight pattern. The taming and the transformation of the structural repetition compulsion can free me from being tossed from one opposite to another, from flight to fight, back and forth and forth and back.[60] If Anna's and my relating pattern

---

[60] According to the latest brain research, the neurons in the brain change in response to the external environment. If one does not feel safe, for example, the amygdala, the primitive part of the brain, takes over from the frontal cortex, the area of the brain responsible for rational thought. The amygdala tells us there is a threat and sends messages to the body in the form of increased adrenaline and cortisol. The body responds by fighting, freezing, or fleeing. This is a survival mechanism. If a threat comes and can be integrated, the amygdala does not take over. If early trauma has repetitively ignited or constellated the amyg-

gradually rearranges itself into an intimate autonomy, there is hope that this interpersonal pattern can reflect back onto this disease's form of torment. And vice versa: The intrapsychic release of the oppositional ons and offs of Parkinson's casts back onto the interpersonal. As a result of this reflective movement, the best scenario would be that a dialectic begins, that a *perpetuum mobile* energy is kicked off, that the ons and the offs become more intimately autonomous with each other.

The joy of being on for me is the experience of a space, a white space, a space of my favorite color. In this white space, I feel colorful, unfettered, and glowing with a light radiating into me and through me. When I am off, I become an object with opened eyes. Parkinson's reigns subjectively supreme. I feel like a marionette on strings; I am turned to stone, a statue unable to move. The space is red. Full of roiling anger, I am rendered helpless, nakedly vulnerable. Inflexible, I tremble with red rage and with fear.

At this time, there is only a one of the two when I am at the mercy of Parkinson's: on or off, white or red. These ones do not relate to each other; they do not play with each other. There is no attunement. The dynamic of a uroboric circle that ensures contact and feedback is but a memory or a hope. An empty chasm yawns between them; the ones are too far apart, or the potential twos disappear when they meet. And again, there is only a lonely one. There is no consciousness of a third space, a space where an inherent dynamic flow allows communication: It can be loud, or it can harbor an empathetic silence. It is a space harboring the Trickster, Merkurius, who consists of all conceivable opposites. He is thus quite obviously a duality, but is named a unity in spite of the fact that his innumerable inner contradictions can dramatically fly apart into an equal number of disparate and apparently independent figures. (Jung, 1971, Vol. 13, para. 267)

It is a space of a feisty, engaging energy whispering adamantly: "intimate autonomy." Presently, relentlessly, throughout the days and

---

dala, it is more difficult to "rewire." The discovered plasticity of the brain offers an opening for—at the least—a hiss of hope for redirecting neurons influential in Parkinson's disease!

throughout the nights, I am either red or I am white. I am either on or I am off. In a space devoid of communication. In a wasteland where "the dead men lost their bones…(and) where a current under the sea/picked his bones in whispers" (Eliot, 1922)[61] Alone.

Parkinson's and I are still entrenched in dualism, each in a separate space.

I—we—that is, Parkinson's and I—have not yet been able to know the relating pattern of an intimate autonomy, of a fluid two in a one. We have not yet been launched into the transforming energy of a paradox.

To launch a *coniunctio*, an inaugural unity, an *unus mundus*, which lies behind—and distills—our world of duality, to learn to know a right distance and closeness, is the *quinta essentia* of Anna's and my voyage. At the point of twos becoming also a one—or for that matter, of a one becoming twos—at the point of a static dualistic power battle capitulating to a dynamic liquidity, a flow, a relating pattern is sparked. In this dialectical dance, the one becomes the two; the twos are also the one. And the dance begins.

Anna and I

Looking back now at the last years, I would describe two people working analytically yet with an unmistakable emphasis on the anaclitic, or this therapy's leaning on orientation. Regarding the relating pattern between Anna and me, there is—and has been—a marked quality of mutual respect, a shared humor, as well as a reciprocal willingness to ingest opposite opinions or clashing ways of being. And we are motivated by common interests, by cautious concern, and we are sparked by considerable curiosity.

Anna and I are experiencing a unique, an engagingly terrifying voyage into this dance of intimate autonomy. Without this outside firm

---

[61] To read the relevant portion of The Waste Land, see Appendix A-9.

interpersonal structure of our relationship, we both sense there would be no possibility of individual intrapsychic rearrangement. No hope of setting an underlying foundational relating pattern for all twos and ones. No shedding of an embedded repetition compulsion, no transformational reshaping of intrapsychic entities. Recognizing the significance of our detailed observations, Anna and I discover the play of opposites, of twos, and their key functions in a pattern of relationship. We locate the central importance of words, with necessary spaces in between, which allows structural vibration, syntactical communication. We note the transformational intensity of embedment into fierce waves, which then flow into calm oceanic waters, with their movement and the throes of their process with each other.

Anna and I are a two, a necessary ingredient of an intimate autonomy. Our voyage takes us to the unity of the two, which is simultaneously the separateness of the one. And the dance of this contradiction, of this paradox, of its quickening a spark of something new, a new consciousness, a new life…all these and none alone constitute the fulcrum of the voyage.

These are Anna's and my concerns and conjectures. We have been encouraged by clinical and amplifying sources that reiterate and confirm our hopes and thereby awaken premonitions of unchartered *hisses*.

Vignettes from Anna's and my voyage

A closer glance at the actual dance movements of this voyage, a few clinical vignettes, can help to shed light on what is meant by *dance*. And with the realization that not only with Parkinson's but with any physical illness, or psychological symptom, and a person's ego can result in a dualistic power battle. For example, in an attempt to gain control over anxiety, or depression, the ego tries to be in charge but often fails. The anxiety rages on. The two are locked in a fight/flight rhythm.

Rather than trying for a calibrated attunement, our interest in Parkinson's and me as oppositional twos becomes more differentiated—and more complicated.

Shockingly revealing for me at the beginning of the relationship between Anna and me is the discovery that intimacy—as one possible dance step—harbors for me moments of existential anxiety.

To lose my exclusivity as a one reveals itself as terrifying. Intimacy is to become a one as part of a two. Since my birth and the vertical split, I have felt alone—desperately, defensively separate. And I have been too separate from Anna. During our voyage, I have wanted to be able to allow myself to lean on, to become more dependent on Anna. Not only physically, a condition to which Parkinson's contributes with his magnanimous and concomitant mean-spirited, dominating, and invasive personality. But also psychologically.

When I literally cannot move—usually a prime nighttime feature of this ever-present dance with Parkinson's—Anna becomes my anchor and guide throughout hysterical and painful waves of being sucked in by the undertow of oppositional currents hidden in oceanic depths. Inundated with nightmares of victimization, I feel anxious. I feel caught in a dark underlying turbulence, in spaces of violence and anarchy. Spaces where Rilke's angels hover and wait to destroy. Anna often becomes the receiver of the panicked fury cascading out of a yet unknown depth of my being. Opening to foreign red entities, energies break out suddenly and leave us both trembling.

The following vignette lends an insight into what such a space can contain:

One early morning, after a night of restlessness and little sleep for both of us, a force created by the distance between my base and the surface tears, elicits a reflective response when I interpret one of Anna's remarks as being sarcastically condescending. I feel not-known, not-seen. With the relentlessness of a tsunami, I insist that I am doing so much, while she questions herself not at all. I yell—"I am constantly aware of my need for ego-control: I have to let go; I have to relax my body and turn it inside out. I have to…" I begin to cry. Then I continue to attack: "That is not balanced, even though our relating is one of twos, of opposites…I alone have to do everything, what do you have to change?" At this point, Anna bursts into tears, and the common space sparkles with rage and vulnerability and at the same time, a shared recognition that we both must "keep these things and ponder them in our hearts." (Luke 2:19)

Anna counters that she feels that she has given so much that she cannot offer any more, that she might as well just quit.

Instead of continuing the aggressive word exchange, however, she pauses. She seems to just know what to do and suddenly, instinctually, begins her baby-whispering way of relating: She takes my hands in hers and just holds them…still…just still, in time and in space…just still. Touching. Holding my arms, she begins to rock them slowly, gently, the way calm waves rock a boat. It is a surreal experience; it feels as if a door in me opens and something lost takes this opportunity to reattach to me. As if a porthole long closed and barricaded had opened, water carries this entity through to me: my infant self, just born, placed on a slippery weighing scale and put into a room by herself. The door is shut.

This passionate, tiny being is the entity who is reached through Anna's baby-whispering, through her sensate touching, through her calm and consistent relating. Through her physical and her psychological presence contacting and rocking me, Anna appears to break through barriers. A regression cannot be planned. It suddenly just happens. Or not. Anna seems to shatter a small section of the frozen, structured repetition compulsion of being only—and safely— a one defensively countermanding intimacy.

Anna rocks my arms slowly, the world opens up to a space of slow continual gentle waves and drops of water caressing, touching my skin, confirming my existence and promising a continuity of care and closeness, and of safety. I feel the slight tremor of a new relationship pattern; from a great distance I hear the resounding swirling of bubbles of joy, and for the first time, I gradually sense a central bedrock of organizational firmness. I comprehend a life without the ubiquitous free-floating anxiety, without the ever-prevalent expectation of sliding off. I can sense a whiff of free-falling instead of resorting to the familiar fight/flight repetition compulsion. Or resorting to yet another defensive technique known to me, but not consciously, until recently reading about it: that of freezing. A third way of avoiding contact, of refusing intimacy, both intrapsychic and interpersonal—as usual.

All of a sudden, I see the opposites of the base and the tip of the breaking wave connecting to each other, relating to each other in their dance between the dense oceanic water flow and the joyful cascading freed drops, a dance of relationship, of knowing each other, not of desperate defensive separation. A dance without the ever-threatening devouring chasm of anxiety. I feel an anticipation of being anchored to myself! I can imagine me, myself being a two—or a more than two-—indwelling in a one. I can feel the movement, back and forth, toward… and away. While Anna rocks my arms back and forth, and forth and back, I can feel the rhythm, the ancient pulse of life and death connecting.

All of this is a mirror of the now even firmer relating pattern with Anna. A mirror of oppositional attunement. A relating pattern of intertwining ones with twos, with dance steps separating and connecting in ancient rhythms of fuguelike structures and teasing notes of winsome beauty.

Along with this new freedom to depend on Anna and the dialectically paradoxical gain in autonomy, I note distinctly another essential feature of our voyage: a sweet and sour loss, the sacrifice, of exclusive will and ego energy.[62] Or perhaps a more appropriate description would be to say my desperate need for ego control trickles away gradually. Not knowing that the base for my ego, that this newly won relationship can hold, the familiar anxiety often slips in, and the wave often breaks. When this happens, any relating or touching between the strawberry-blonde infant and my worldly ego dissolves. Any new bridge forged in the moment of Anna's touch collapses. And once again I am off.

---

[62] An experience Ahab was to never know.

John and I

My journey with Parkinson's has become our journey; my voyage into an intimate autonomy becomes my husband John's journey also; any transformation of consciousness on my part reflects back to him. And vice versa. These are inevitabilities if twos are also ones.

My husband's caring for me during nights of offness, during days of fight/flight and freezing, during moments when I cannot dance anymore—for the most part—are examples of a fusion through the soul. For this I am grateful.

At the onset of our relationship, the opposites are so far apart that any recognition of a soul connection is mute. One poignant memory has us sitting in an Indian restaurant in Frankfurt. We had met for the first time two weeks earlier. Since then, we have spent all of our free time together. In the restaurant the food is fantastic, the margaritas are copious and strong, the conversations reveal wavelengths of light, of communicative vessels.

We are both feeling the unusual rapport. We are both in a space of cataclysmic soul potentialities, when John looks into my eyes and says: "Meredith, I love you."

I am shocked! After living so long in Germany, I had become unconsciously conscious of the immanent quality of the word—and especially of such a word as *love*. After thanking him profusely for such a compliment, I say to him: "You must mean *agape*." His reaction I will never forget. He asks: "What in the fuck is *agape*?"

Two years later, in 1997, I was given the diagnosis of Parkinson's disease. I had flown to Canada in June to marry John—at least that had been the plan. Now I know that since no man would be willing to spend the rest of his life with a disease, I plan to enjoy the days with him in Montreal and then return to my life in Germany. Sitting across from him on a sunny day in a 1950s hamburger restaurant, I told him with tears dripping down my cheeks, that I have Parkinson's disease. Without a second's hesitation, John reaches over to take my hand and says:

"Through sickness and through health, till death do us part." The delicious North American hamburger remains uneaten.

The dragonfly and I

To reconnect with a key interpersonal and intrapsychic partner besides Anna and John, whose attachment are central to my transmutation, I want to recall my spirit animal, the dragonfly. I want to remind Anna and me of its presence. And I want to remind the dragonfly of us. Its instinctual consciousness, its differentiated manner of seeing and of moving open a dimension iconic in its mystical and creative quality of presence, unique in its influence on me, and singularly and incomparably contributive to my potential harvesting of a new form of life. The dragonfly imparts a speed and a stillness, an oppositional attunement—or a syzygian Hegelian synthesis—daring me to undertake this journey. And the dragonfly lends me its special kind of hope to try. (And to consciously swallow a possible swing into its opposite of no-hope.) I recall the equanimity of the *hiss* and even with the newness of unfamiliar, potentially treacherous waters I am determined to try.

In a later chapter, I have recorded in more personal detail, clinical vignettes and encounters with the dragonfly that suggest a mysterious connection. These stories reaffirm the eerie exclusivity of a relationship with a spirit animal.

Ahab and Moby Dick

In an earlier chapter I used the narrative device of the fairy tale to exemplify relating patterns that are too close or too distant. With Herman Melville's *Moby Dick*, I use another kind of narrative to highlight the danger of a relating pattern that is too close, too entangled.

In this internationally acclaimed 19th-century novel, Melville plays with the notions of opposition and of alchemy. The protagonist, Captain Ahab, fails to consciously experience the darkness of the alchemical *nigredo*, the beginning of the transformative opus, while Ishmael, the narrator of the drama, bears this alchemical process. Melville describes Ishmael as being "surrounded by blocks of blackness" (Melville, 1847/1967, p. 18). Later in the novel, this subprotagonist of *Moby Dick* remarks: "I felt a melting within. ... The soothing savage [Queequeg] has redeemed it [my heart and my head]" (Melville, p. 53). This alchemical *dissolutio* is akin to our regression and the story of the well.

As a contrast (and as a unity) the *nigredo* occurs at the end of the novel. It is left open as to whether or not Ahab's death is an experience of a single one, or if Moby Dick dies with the captain of the sinking ship. Melville leaves us to ponder (similar to the ending of *Faust*, where Goethe leaves the reader also with riddles or paradoxes). Ishmael concludes the narrative of the voyage. He reports that he "was drawn to the closing vortex. ... Round and round, then, and ever contracting towards the button-like *black* bubble at the axis of that slow wheeling circle . . . I did revolve. Till, gaining that vital center, the black bubble upwards burst; and now liberated by reason of its cunning spring, and, owing to its great buoyancy, rising from the sea with great force, the coffin life-buoy shot lengthwise from the sea, fell over and floated by my side. ... On the second day, a sail drew near, nearer, and picked me up at last" (Melville, p. 470).[63]

The regressive space

Separation or entanglement, a too-distant or too-close relating pattern, is the syntactical dualistic structure that Anna and I hope to dissolve on

---

[63] The name Ishmael is biblical in origin and means "God shall hear." In Genesis 16:1-16; 17:18-25; 15:9-217, Ishmael is banished to the "wilderness of Beer-sheba," while the narrator of Moby Dick wanders, in his own words, in the "wilderness of waters." In the Bible, Ishmael is saved by his own name when in the desert a well of water suddenly appears. In Moby Dick, likewise, only Ishmael escapes the sinking of the ship and that by a margin so narrow as to seem miraculous. This "secondary figure" is portrayed as being able to give of himself without losing himself, e.g., in the relationship with Queequeg [intimacy] and he can be vulnerable, e.g., with the wind and the waves on a sea journey [autonomy].

our voyage. In a culminating full nothingness, a wilderness revealed by a regression, a restructuring or reorganization can begin to form. The function of the regression encompasses the form. And vice versa. Alchemically, adhering to a uroboric circular trajectory, the form and the function are a *dissolutio* and a *coagulatio* rhythmically interchanging reciprocity. The dynamic living quality of this two in one of our intimate autonomy, instead of the more common static stuckness of a dualistic structure, is the *telos* of the voyage.

Beginning at the moment of my birth, my crying is loud and passionate. Neither the nurses nor my mother feels able to withstand the intensity. Instead of rocking me or touching me, they decide to *let me develop my lungs* while separated from them and from the other newborns who were "good babies": They are all quiet. The door is shut. I am placed on a slippery weighing machine without any containing perimeters. Alone with my fears, my anxiety, and my screams.

This tiny being has but a minuscule ego. She is unable to hold the tension of the betrayal of the womb's safety and then the slide to another world where there is an emptiness filled with pain and anxiety. Her body retains the memory of these moments while her mind, her psyche, her soul dissociates and forgets.

This is the space I have to return to. I have to experience this terror once again. Only there will a reorganization be possible.

I want to repeat the story of Jung's patient, of her dream and the well:

I was in a well and couldn't get out. Scrambling towards the top, I became aware that a fire had been set under me, that the flames were becoming higher and hotter. I was desperate to get out. My hands were scratched and bleeding from trying to pull myself up on the brick sides of the well. I finally reached the top of the well and, hanging onto the brick rim, I yelled for Jung to help me. I heard his footsteps; he came up to the edge of the well. Laughing, Jung said, "You don't want out, you want in!" And he pushed me down into the flames.

I recall the words of Jesus in the Apocryphon of John. The words were something like: "If I am a lamp for you, then you can see me; if I am a mirror for you, then you know me." And I wonder at the depth of a mirror compared to a lamp. We must have a *mirrored* experience to connect to before any reorganization can take place.

We have to assume that Dr. Jung's analytic work with his patient has enabled her to *remember*; that is, to reassociate the trauma experienced, to reconnect it with her body and her mind, and to have had the intense intimate autonomous work, the interpersonal, the mirroring work, with Jung that enables her to know that she is known, perceived, and safe. This structural, syntaxical perimeter, this containment is now digested and has become a centripetal force, the *form has realized its function*. The repetition compulsive mistrust and expectation of betrayal yield to an introjection of a relating pattern of just enough distance and closeness and just enough containment.

The immediate experience of existential anxiety contributes to my experience of falling down the well, a razor-sharp awareness of unconscious depths and their hidden, shadowy supremacy. I can now recognize when anxiety stimulates the waves to breakage and when Parkinson's slides through and the exclusive physical experience of illness grabs and claims me. In both cases, I am off. Being able to consciously differentiate anxiety from physical symptoms demands a fine-tuning of the relationship between mind and body. And between the conscious and the unconscious. Between the ego as choreographer of conscious dance steps and anxiety as reassembled signs of pirouettes hidden in the unconscious. And I know now that most experiences of harmony, balance, or even serenity resulting from this dance of teardrops and cascading oceanic water, that their equilibrium first depends on taming torrents of terrifying anxiety. This taming—as in Antoine de Saint-Exupery's 1943 story of the prince and the fox in *The Little Prince*—requires patience, time, and presence. And touch.

A clinical vignette

The taming in this expedited process of allowing myself to sacrifice at the least a modicum of ego-control peaks in yet another night of terror.

In this same night, however, I am a participant in an astonishingly resolute attachment. I want to relate this experience in some detail. This is for me a core occurrence on our voyage. It begins with this dream:

I am in a room, but a room on top of moving water. My parents are in the rectangular boat-room with me. On the left side, my mother keeps wanting to slide out of the room into the water. Anticipating this, I constantly watch the door to ensure that it is closed. At the same time, my father keeps trying to slide open the wall, his door, to view a violent scene outside on the street. There are men lying on the street, killed by people who are now trying to enter our house boat. Instead of protecting us, my father wants to get out and view everything from the outside. At the same time, I am frantically trying to keep my balance because the undulating water is sliding us all back and forth. I concentrate on keeping the doors shut from the inside and also I am determinedly desperate to avert the threat from the outside. It seems an impossible task. Then I realize I am losing my balance; I am losing control over my body! But just at that moment of panic, a woman with Anna's body yet with black hair demonstrates that she can slip out and into the water and pull herself back up into our boat. Her ability to not be stuck anywhere, her confident dynamic sliding, helps me to feel safer. But upon waking, I remain primarily in my tense terror and in the repetitive and frantic acting out.

Throughout the dream—in this other world yet through a diaphanous membrane, a mirror of the dream scene—I know I am slipping off the bed. Overcome by my hysterical features, I am continually sure that any minute I will lose control and actually slip off the bed. In a panic, I scream Anna's name. With an inner strength and autonomous vulnerability like the woman with black hair in my dream, she comes immediately. But then she keeps pushing me into my terror. Like Jung, but without the laughter, she repetitively chants: "Slip, Meredith, slip!"

Later, discussing the dream and the night's experience, Anna and I surmise that the dream reflects my earliest memory of being in the room by myself after birth, perhaps placed and left on the slippery baby scale. There is not a conscious figment of a memory of that primal experience, but the feeling of that night and its horror has remained with me my whole life. This time, however, I do not get stuck on the scale. I do not get stuck in the fear. This time I do slip, I do let go of ego control, and I do get at the least a slight glimpse of dwelling in my body, or, to use Winnicott's term, *personalisation* (Winnicott, 1971, pp. 41-42).[64] Perhaps some layer of skin could finally form. A structural agency affecting inside and outside spaces, a physical presence I can trust. This membrane affords me a form, a gestalt, an identity.

With the birth of this secure structure, plus the corollary of a relative softening of ego-control, I find myself more attached. More attached to Anna, attached to my body, attached to a strongly defined drop of a centripetal distilled center.

Yet I am now acquainted with a new space of survival, a space in-between rather than split off, a space together with—rather than separate from—a once-upon-a-time foreign space I can now taste and smell. A space where I can touch another human being. A space inhabited by some other power, perhaps a dragonfly nymph in me, who doesn't need ego control, who can whirl through the water and dart over and under the waves. Perhaps guided more by instinct…perhaps it does not know the terror engendered by the fear of being alone, the fear of slipping off anything…perhaps if I breathe more and deeply, my nostrils will redden, and the timid newborn will feel the beauty of the breath of the one and of the two—a biological reality already known to her in the womb.

Rilke's words and their oppositional attunement suddenly emerge once again: "For what strikes us as beauty is nothing/ but all we can bear of a terror's beginning,/and we admire it so, because it calmly disdains/to destroy us. Every angel strikes terror" (Rilke, trans. Oswald, 1992, p. 26).[65]

---

[64] "The basis for this indwelling is a linkage of motor and sensory and functional experience with infant's new state of being…a limiting membrane…between the infant's 'me' and 'not-me'…Without [(this linkage]…a relationship to shared reality is difficult because instinct experiences, which are an essential basis for this relationship, cannot be felt with the full intensity of total involvement. And total involvement inheres regression back to the original trauma."

[65] "Denn das Schoene ist nichts/als des Schrecklichen Anfang, den wir noch grade ertragen,/ und wir bewundern es so, weil es gelassen verschmaeht,/ uns zu zerstören. Ein jeder Engel ist schrecklich."

Part Three

A child of light is born

Ultimately, recapitulating, we recognize that our voyage has to apprehend that this book's emphasis on patterns of relating is structurally concerned with opposites. They are the twos. The twos of Parkinson's and me, of Anna and me, of my husband and me, of the dragonfly and me, of Ahab and the white whale, of white and red—ad infinitum. And we are dealing with the relationships between these twos, with our ultimate concern being their ability to slide into and out of the one. When the twos prance into a paradox and gleefully leave at least part of the ego behind, their original structural components are opposites. The concentration is to find an oppositional attunement in an autopoietic synthetic relating pattern that intrinsically harbors the dynamic dialectic of closeness and distance, be it between persons, words, energies, or tending the invasion of a disease.

To embark on our passage, we have to voyage into a regressive, a dusky space, an empty-nothingness space, open to Rilke's terror-eliciting angels. A space of potential prospects of death, of ego fragmentation, yet teeming with angels who also ensure survival, who disdain to destroy. A space where dependency can transform into autonomy, where first, however, the pain and the anxiety felt in a regressive encounter can be overwhelming. Endemic to this regressive space, indicative of the unveiling of hitherto hidden shadows, the repetition compulsion to vertically split is unconsciously, as well as consciously, alluring.

On the other hand, the yearning for the experience of being known, the existentially experienced need to be a one of a two and its betrayal is the embedded repetition compulsive structure of what Freud calls a *reaction formation*; that is, I get stuck in the opposite of what I really desire. Indeed, I have mirrored my mother's not letting me in by separating myself in the identification with the frozen cold separateness of the Snow Queen. If I remain separate and get there first, then I can't be hurt. A primal repetitive defense mechanism. Counter-phobic! Very successful!

127

Doing the opposite of what I consciously want is crazy. Indeed. Nonetheless, this intrapsychic boomerang energy and its repetitive scaffolding throughout my life has held me, it has contained me. This structural repetition compulsion has helped me to remain sane. In moments of regression during which the shedding of this structure has been noted, I feel as if I am in a foreign country and do not know the language.

Our voyage does not feel like a fiery hunt, like Ahab's obsessive desire to find the whale. We have embarked with curiosity, with Anna's generosity, and with deep suffering. Our consciousness sets the course; we both know that the preverbal infant and I belong together, that we are the two in one. We know that this mirrored, reflected intrapsychic unity can assume form—if and when Anna and I, interpersonally, can enter into and can hold the relating pattern of an intimate autonomy.

We know now that she and I together can rock me, we can rock my body and me, into a new relatedness, into a new pattern with the other. This rocking is mirrored and reflects on intrapsychic patterns also. Included is the manner of my relating to Parkinson's. We can liquefy into our two-in-one syzygical unity. Parkinson's can accompany me on Melville's white steed, a horse whose red and white, whose opposites—each in its single actuality—belong together. Like the white steed Melville describes, we can gather together our combined strengths and sacrifice the need for a *powder power*, the putative strength derived from dualistic combat. Instead of one against one, our slides of twos into ones, our dance of opposites, reflects the red and white *coniunctio* of Melville's horse:

> Most famous in our Western annals and Indian traditions is that of the *White* Steed of the Prairies...the White Steed... with warm nostrils *reddening* through his cool milkiness; in whatever aspect he presented himself, always to the bravest Indians he was the object of trembling reverence and awe. (Melville, 1847/1967, p.165)

A voyage of transformation can change elements in the deepest structures of matter while floating in psychic obfuscations bewildering the most enlightened. Opposite currents clash, waves break until a base at the bottom of the ocean attaches itself to drops on the surface and the voyage transforms from a desperate fiery hunt to a soft undulating cruise. Anna and I remark at the beauty of the red sunset dipping into the white colorless water until both attach, and the world becomes a reflection of Indra's net and of its knots of many hues. We know now that separation is not real, but we know also that separation has its fugitive moments in the process of a union of opposites. And we know that a ride on the white steed, a ride on the oceanic waves of the paradox of an intimate autonomy, can be both exhilarating and terrifying. We know also that it is—partly at least—a matter of choice.

Anna has left once again. I am pregnant with the experience of a new space, a space replete with that momentary experience of attachment, of an *indwelling in my body*, of a child of light, and of a safe space when Anna is near. After a hiatus of five weeks, she returns and the cruise—or the voyage—continues. Perhaps this time it will take place in a distant yet close silvery-white glade of light whose speed is the only constant in the world and leaves red sparks in its tracks. Perhaps reflecting the reattachment of my hitherto split-off infant base and me, a two in one—a unified duality between Parkinson's on and his off—can assume a liquid yet firm form (Jung, 1984, Bd. 14, para. 42). [66] We do not question the possibility; nor do we expect an answer. It is a voyage.

I used to water ski, skipping along the surface of the ocean's waters…

---

[66] "Alchemy has its own scintilla. First and foremost the scintilla is the fiery center of the earth… everything originates from this center and nothing can be born unless it comes from this source…. If one becomes conscious due to the relationship with this light, any trace of doubt disappears, and without any difficulty, one will be able to 'know' this magnetic point which emits the paradoxical rays of the sun and of the earth concomitantly." German translation: "die Alchemie hat ihre Scintilla. Sie ist zunaechst das feurige Erdzentrum….'Alle Dinge naemlich haben ihren Ursprung in dieser Quelle, und gar nichts in der ganze Welt wird geboren ausser durch dieser Quelle…wenn einer vom Licht der Natur erleuchtet wird, so verschwindet der Nebel vor seinen Augen, und ohne Beschwer vermag er den Punkt unseres Magneten zu erblicken, welcher dem doppelten Strahlenzentrum der Sonne und der Erde entspricht."

Molt 12: The dynamic dialectic of play—Galatea

Our voyage continues. Different from the journey of Ahab and the whale, where the relating pattern remains embedded in dualism, Anna and I are in a ship, harboring hope for a different relationship, in a relating pattern that opens to a third space of play.[67] Here, we as two can drift into—and out of —moments of being one: a pattern we call an intimate autonomy, a relating pattern shattering and dispersing the static quality of a nonattuned dualism, a nondynamic dialectical meeting, a disconnected opposition—or its opposite: a projective identification. An intimate autonomous relating pattern is relevant to—and worthy of note for— any twos or more. A pattern whose gradual and intricate realization generates a fundamental core of this book. A cornerstone of the dignity of the *hiss* and the hope/no hope, as well as of Anna and of me, of the dragonfly and me, and, of course, of Parkinson's and me.

In my relationship with Parkinson's currently, the two contending forces of this disease, the ons and the offs, are still catapulting me from one opposite to the other. The third space rarely opens for us. During the night, for the most part, Parkinson's disease renders me off. A physical paralysis. A Galatea condition.

In Ovid's *Metamorphoses*, in the 10th book, there is a tale of creativity, of beauty and of love. And of transformation.

Galatea

The artist, Pygmalion, labors long and devotedly, daily sculpting with his hands and with his fingers the most exquisite statue of a woman. With each

---

[67] As a contrasting relating pattern, Herman Melville's Moby Dick depicts the captain of the ship, Ahab, desperately hunting for the white whale. The whale had cost him his leg; revenge became Ahab's sole goal. The relating pattern clinically is projective identification, a dualistic form of projection and then identification. In an intimate autonomy, a third becomes inevitable due to the spark of the paradox: the space of the hiss. As I've pointed out, this "third" is actually not a third; but rather, it is a one composed of the dynamic quality of the paradoxical twos. It is new space of consciousness—the space of a syzygy.

caress her beauty and her perfection increase; with each invasive thrust of his tools the stone reveals more and more of its truth. Upon completion, Pygmalion steps back. He distances himself from his task and observes that he and the white marble stone have forged together a true work of art, a form beyond his own skill, a statue of such deep beauty, that he knows it to have touched an eternal chord. Astounded, he realizes her beauty is timeless. He also recognizes that he has fallen in love.

A marble statue, a beautiful woman white as snow. A passionate love. He kisses her lips, he takes her in his arms, he dresses her in rich robes and lays red roses at her snow-white feet. Despite daily and nightly offerings of heartfelt homage, she remains lifeless. Pygmalion becomes hopelessly, wretchedly despondent. He weeps copious tears. He prays. He prostrates himself at the temple where incense burns, at the temple of the Goddess of Love, at Aphrodite's temple.

Aphrodite is interested in someone different, in someone who is a new kind of lover: a man who can truly love another and still remain faithful to himself. And as she herself is born of violence, she is drawn by the sculptor's aggressively creative manner of bringing this woman into existence, of his hammer and of his sharp cutting tools. She is moved by his tears. Aphrodite feels an affinity with his sculpture, for while she herself was born of Nature's waters, Pygmalion's statue emerges out of Nature's stone.

Unaware of his own special allure for the Goddess, Pygmalion begins his usual evening ritual upon his arrival at home. Still despondent, yet marveling and loving the white marble body, he bestows his usual kiss on the statue's full and shapely pale lips. He caresses her cold, hard but perfectly formed face. Is it self-deception or are the lips warm and soft? He touches her arms, her shoulders. They feel like wax melting in the sun. He clasps her white wrist; he sees red blood pulsing there! With unutterable gratitude and joy he puts his arms around his love and sees her smile and blush.

He names her Galatea; their daughter they name Paphos, from whom the island later takes its name.

The figure on the cover portrays metaphorically the author when Parkinson's "freezes" her. Concurrently, the stature represents the mythical Galatea.

Upside-down play

During the night I become a statue and cannot move. Lying in bed, I often think: "The only part of my body that remains accessible to my control is my breath." So, I take deep breaths, as deep as I can. Sometimes I notice a slight movement in my stomach. A slight gasp of *chi* energy. And hope flutters (while no-hope copes). Breath becomes a kind of reified pipeline, a coagulated umbilical cord, from the outside to the inside of me. The inevitable relating between the inside and the outside is confirmed through the breath and—like that of a baby and a mother—I know that I am each and both. I could know something in addition; I intuit, I sense something of a key to a secret garden, a key I have not yet found.

Last night, breathing, I note a huge flutter inside. Hope moves up into my thoughts: "If I could just flip over the wellspring of control, from the outside to the inside! I could imagine that my body would receive commands from the inside instead of the outside, from an entity and a space not yet familiar! Instead of my well-known and used outside ego. Perhaps then Aphrodite would come and free my real self. Perhaps then I—like Galatea—could melt like wax in the sun."

D. W. Winnicot published a book, *Playing and Reality*, in the early 1970s, in which the self is portrayed as often caught in the tension of inner and outer realities, of their being "welded" together (Winnicott, 1971, p. 13). I know his writings…but then, instead of continuing along his trajectory of the inevitable embedment of these two realities and their potential opening between: into his *intermediate area of experience*—(the space of Goethe's attuned opposition or our third space harboring and nurturing a further step into a new intimate autonomy)—my thoughts fall into the kitchen and land on my mother's recipe for a delicious upside-down ginger bread:

Part Three

Gingerbread Upside-down Cake

1 cup sifted flour
½ teaspoon baking soda
¼ teaspoon salt
2 teaspoons cinnamon
1 teaspoon ginger
¼ teaspoon nutmeg
1 egg, slightly beaten
5 tablespoons dark brown sugar
¼ cup molasses
½ cup buttermilk
¼ cup shortening, melted
¼ cup butter
1/3 cup firmly packed brown sugar

Mix and sift flour, baking soda, salt and spices. (I always increase the amount of spices and add ground cloves and allspice). Combine egg, sugar, molasses, buttermilk, and shortening. Gradually add flour mixture, stirring until mixed. Beat vigorously about 1 minute, or until smooth. Put the greased shallow pan in which it is to be baked on a low burner: add butter and brown sugar. Melt them together and add pears or another fruit you may select. Pour batter over the fruit. Bake in a pre-heated 350-degree Fahrenheit oven for about 35 to 40 minutes.

Let it cool for about 10 minutes. And now comes the challenge: Hold the pan just right and then flip it over. The inside becomes the outside!

Why and how do I think of mother's upside-down gingerbread? What can the recipe have to do with Parkinson's disease and me? Or, for that matter, with the myth of Galatea? Or even if the gingerbread adds a hitherto unknown ingredient and bakes itself to yet another level, does this really entertain a relevance to Goethe, to Ahab and Moby Dick, to us? Where is the missing key?

Winnicott found a path out of the welded *inner and outer*, out of specified constitutive parts: He writes about the "*third* area of human

THE HISS OF HOPE

living, one neither inside the individual nor outside in the world of shared reality. [This] intermediate area of experience starts with children playing." Winnicott emphasizes that play stands at the interface of the outer and the world of inner psychological process. He writes: "Into this play area the child gathers objects or phenomena from external reality and uses these in the service of some sample derived from inner or personal reality...." (Winnicott, 1971, p. 51).

The philosopher and clinical psychologist, J. W. Jones, reminds us that the child uses toys and other objects that she invests with special meaning. This creative capacity, however, continues to develop after the toys have been put aside. Toys are the catalysts of the creative capacity. When (these) toys recede into the background, there remains the residue of the inventiveness that generates art and the curiosity that drives science, that is the capacity to create culture. (Jones, 2002, p. 45)

I am playing with the gingerbread! Unconsciously, I am trying to contact Aphrodite and elicit her inventiveness in my inner reality! Pygmalion is playing with Galatea in a third space when he brings her roses, when he dresses her in rich robes, when he kisses her lips. Only then does Aphrodite intervene and make her real in an external reality.

Is *playing* the key that opens our third space? In this intermediate third space, where the tension inherent in the dualism of inner and outer, between objectivity and subjectivity, between power and disempowerment, does play melt a solidified duality into a liquid dialectic, into fluid patterns of relating?

Relating, or play, demands space and time. It also demands an extrication from total ego control, a disengagement from a place of power. This third space is conceptual; it is an empty space sans *telos*, a space in which creation can begin. There is no ascribed form, or function, or structure. It is real and not real; it is, and it isn't. In the ancient Hindu text, the *Brahma Sutras*, the reality of this third space is explained: "Whenever we claim something is unreal, it is in reference to something real." In the myth, Galatea becomes real! This third space harbors a haven of transformational mist (Winnicott's residue of inventiveness), which hovers in an alchemical laboratory focusing on the essences of physical materials and their potential transmutation. Alchemy is not magic. It is cryptic creativity.

When a child begins to play—like Pygmalion—she "invests chosen external phenomena with dream meaning and feeling," Winnicott avers. He continues:

> I am therefore studying the substance of illusion, that which is allowed to the infant, and which in adult life is inherent in art and religion, and yet becomes the hallmark of madness when an adult puts too powerful a claim on the credulity of others, forcing them to acknowledge a sharing of illusion that is not their own. Winnicott, 1971, p. 51)

Etymologically, the word *play* finds some of its roots in the Latin *ludus* (the play) and *ludere* (to play). In other cultures, the primal roots for play likewise denote movement (Huizinga, 1949/1955).

Perhaps one can allude to the ingredients in the gingerbread as playing with each other while being baked. The movement in the oven of the mists of transformation is also at work. Separated multiple constituent parts are transmuted into a one. When I eat the one, with close concentration, I can savor simultaneously the each of the many.

How can one word, namely the word *play*, rooted in nature, in the movement of the wind and the waves, be a spin-off of an alchemical process and at the same time be frivolous and aerial? How can the source of play be descriptive of the behavior of animals and at the same time be the performance of a sacred act? Can we really regard the preparation and the baking of gingerbread as play? Perhaps paradox is playful in its seductive movement, beguiling in its cryptic creativity, in its very mystery: *Faust* ends with words of paradox, perplexing riddles chosen by Goethe to seduce and delight the reader, to compel the reader—and future readers—to wrestle, to play, with the mystery of the discordant words for generation after generation (Trunz, 1996, p. 464). [68]

Perhaps the inner goddess of love, Aphrodite, can touch an outer moment of love, perhaps a third-space dance of pulsating movement, and perhaps this dynamic dialectic of play can spark Parkinson's core oppositional ons and offs and with the aqueous sibilance of the *hisses* of hope introduce a watery continuum, a flow-*play*. Perhaps this is the key to a secret garden, where a movement disorder finds itself vibrating and flourishing as a dance of change and fluctuation rather than being trapped in a relating pattern of dualistic desiccated opposition. Or in a *disorder* of unsculpted Galatea marble.

Molt 11: The transmutation of the ice mirror

Connectivity, movement, reality, and apophasis (the Trickster archetype, Merkurius, rhetorical irony) are attributes of what I call *the third space*. With these four traits in mind, I will try to impart further qualities of this space and of this journey by illuminating relevant experiences of the next sequence of the voyage.

Anna returns to Edmonton for six weeks after a hiatus of two months. In these two months, I am able to discern certain changes in attitude perhaps or in physical reactive responses…or in both of these; a weaving in and out of the two trajectories of mind and body, which are also one, a now familiar experience of an intimate autonomy. There are new spaces and byproducts, results of the first part of the voyage.

---

[68] [I ended Faust with paradoxes] "so that everything together remains a riddle, which is going to keep everything a mystery. For centuries this will delight and at the same time it will confuse and keep people fascinated" [Author's translation]. (…damit alles zusammen ein offenbares Raetsel bleibe, die Menschen fort und fort ergoetze und ihnen zu schaffen macht.)

Faust's concluding words: [Author's translation]: Everything transient /Is merely a mirror./The things abstruse /Become soon clear,/The nameless/ Here, it is always sung/ The eternal feminine/ lures us on. (Alles Vergaengliche/ ist nur ein Gleichnis:/ Das Unzulaengliche ,/ Hier wird's Ereignis;/ Das Unbeschreibliche/ Hier ist's getan;/ Das Ewig-Weibliche/Zieht uns hinan.)

Part Three

After Anna left to return to Germany, I note that I can stand my ground in situations where previously anxiety would have prompted an off period, where Parkinson's could slip through the wave-breakage and would have gleefully assumed command, where the repetition compulsion of *feeling at the mercy of* would have asserted its sardonically scathing hegemony over me once again. The present feeling, however, is not a loss of ego control; it feels softer than that. Perhaps more in the manner, not of a submission, but of a surrender. Currently, my reaction to lack of control is not primarily to slide along the structure of fight or flight, but both consciously and unconsciously to *attach* to an entity or to the *solidity of a space* in me. Often now I experience a subsequent strengthened acceptance and a quiver of curiosity, a "sense of self, a sense of wholeness, even a sense of unity with other living beings" (Ghent, 1990, p. 111). A participation in something new.

At the beginning of this part of the voyage, a clear and concise image appears and persists in reasserting its presence again and again: a dolphin has replaced Ahab's whale. There is also a cat and the infant me, all under water, swimming around trying to break through a sheet of ice that would allow us to gain access to the *outside* me. We can talk with each other; we can touch each other. My new sense of wholeness is anchored in an experience of something solid within me as well as a knowledge of belonging to the collective outside. The ice is a wall, a wall between, a double-sided mirror reflecting the inside and the outside. This ice mirror freezes the inside and outside in their respective duality, corroborating their oppositional character.[69] *Inside* and *outside* are twos with no possibility of sliding into and out of a one.

At the same time—because of the inevitability of light's velocity—the mirror simultaneously captures movement. And because my breath is *magic air,* it elicits shapes to "rise up out of mist and vapour" (Trunz, 1996, *Faust I Dedication*, lines 6-8). Enlivened by my breath, the mirror

---

[69] The image of ice mirror depicts a clinical reification of a vertical split, an attempt by the psyche to defend against being overwhelmed. For me, it protects me from being engulfed by anxiety. For further elucidation of a vertical split, see Molt 2.

becomes opened to the space of a "primal wilderness" of playing and of truth (Giegerich, 1998, pp. 205-207), and to the time of "the twilight which we can learn to understand only through inoffensive empathy, but which too much clarity dispels" (Jung, 1982, Bd. 13, para. 199). While the ice solidifies hostility, *the wind and the waves*, the movement of playing, are captured and interiorized by the mirror, enjoyed by the mirror. The ice shatters. The mirror revels in its freedom of movement. Astounded, the mirror staggers and, prismatically, light breaks into myriad colors. The mirror witnesses its own opening up, its transformation from inanimate to animate. Or from immobile to a mobility. And all this it reflects out. A paradox. Yet clearly a key.

The movement

Last night, once again, I cannot move. I am a statue. I lie still and envision the whale transmuted to a dolphin. The dolphin and I begin to play. I ride on its back, we sway back and forth and forth and back in the water. We are gently held and impelled by the moving water. During one of the sleep phases of this night, I have a significant dream:
I am challenged to climb a tree, a strange tree, a tree that looks like a needle, no branches. There are footholds like on a cliff to hang on to. As well as to place my foot into. The challenge is to play with my anxiety and to try to reach the top of the tree. It seems to take ages. I am so proud of myself when I finally reach the top. But then suddenly I realize that I have yet to go down, a maneuver that could be far more anxiety-provoking than the ascent. At that moment this thought climaxes with a rush of adrenaline. But then the tree begins to oscillate, to sway gently back and forth, and forth and back. A soothing rush of tranquility spreads itself throughout my body. The tree slowly, gradually lowers its tip as if to incline its head in a gesture of empathy—and sets me gracefully onto the ground. I get off.

The movement, the soothing rocking of the tree recalls Anna's previous slow, gentle rocking of my arms, the movement of the good-enough mother. The dream plus the dolphin—both inside entities—invite me to play. On the outside the emphasis on the physically experienced gentle rhythmic rocking seems to have coagulated in my blood and become etched in my cells (Oenning-Hodgson, 2007, p. 48). My movements *outside* during the days when I am on are mirroring the swaying softness and—when I catch myself smiling—I know that inside, the dolphin and the not-I are playing in the water. That the ice mirror has become permeable and has opened, I also know. And that this third space has jostled the inside and the outside of the ice mirror further and further apart until there is space between them. Perhaps in time, perhaps at twilight, the ice mirror will liquefy like wax, and the three spaces: the ice, the mirror, and the third space—all of which are there and not-there—will all be open to flow into and flow out of each other. And become one. And three.

The real

Is this all an illusion? What is real anyway? For Winnicott, life has the quality of reality when one is in touch with the centripetal core of a person. This relationship grants life its anchor. The teddy bear carried around by the small child, the dolphin the not-I ride, the tree in my dream…all these are bridges to my "core," to a *not-me*, to Winnicott's "True Self" (Winnicott, 1971, pp. 51-55). Do they lend my life a sense of security and phenomenological safety? For me, without these symbolic conveyors of energy and connectivity "Life …is a tale/ Told by an idiot, full of sound and fury/ Signifying nothing."[70] In *The Velveteen Rabbit*, the popular children's book by Margery Williams, *real* is "When a child loves you for a long, long time not just to play with but really loves you, then you become Real…. When you are Real you don't mind being hurt." (Williams, 1986, p. 14)

---

[70] Macbeth expresses hopelessness with these words. It comes as a huge relief and indeed as a ray of hope, when confronted by Macduff and the knowledge of doom, he meets his death with fighting words.

The three highlights from the voyage up until now have to do with feeling real: learning to depend on and to use Anna; sacrificing a great deal of willpower and ego-control; and differentiating between Parkinson's and anxiety, both of which would turn me into a statue. I have yet to know the quality of presence of my spirit animal, the dragonfly. At this point I can only sense it and its metamorphoses, its shedding an exoskeleton with each molt, and its gradual transmutation from a nymph to an adult dragonfly. The love that the child feels for the Velveteen Rabbit, the love that Pygmalion feels for Galatea, I am yet unable to sense a similar yearning for the dragonfly. It remains but a notion for me. Nor do I experience or feel trust in its guidance.

Can I trust a notion? You can allow yourself to become dependent, if the other is real enough, to not have to trust. You have to know that even if you were betrayed, you would survive. You can become vulnerable. It would hurt and perhaps be alarming, but you would know to endure this kind of encounter. The sacrifice of some ego-control and willpower belongs likewise to feeling the other as real. If the dragonfly is real, there is a diminished threat in relinquishing ego-control. Curiosity can take over. My desperate need to control diminishes. I wonder what is going to happen with the dragonfly. Why is this rather foreign insect in my life?

The third task, that of distinguishing between anxiety and physical symptoms of Parkinson's, both of which render me off and turn me into a statue, have been transmuted from a *thinking* to an embodied experiential recognition of a way to cope with being off. The attachment with something inside dissolves at least part of the tendency to the dualistic power battle of the stuck opposites of on and off. When I feel the stone statue's immobility, its enveloping descent engulfing me, I have learned to attach to the physical rocking of the tree and to the animated four newborn kittens, images from a recent dream. Also, I can attach to the physical memory of Anna rocking my arms. They command me now. This movement, this playing, this process of attaching to that key core of mine makes me often feel firm, solid, and real.

I know the difference now between feeling real and being unreal. Up until now I have been so busy dealing with anxiety that even the ideal of feeling real has been peripheral. Rather like Parkinson's claiming an almost total absorption during the off periods. After the tree dream and our playing together, I can consciously climb an anxiety attack for the first time in my life. Afterward,I feel dizzy, sort of like being in a new country, perhaps like culture shock, not knowing what to do or how to act. Sort of like wandering around in a dream. Like being *inside* instead of *outside*…or perhaps more like being in both at the same time. And again, now, the incredible new softness, the softness of body movements, the softness of feeling silky, the softness of time. And of space. No right-angle corners, just flowing. The softness of a new relating pattern, like Luce Irigaray's "'much love to you'…a way of expressing love that is irresistible yet seeks to be non-appropriative." (Irigaray, 1996 and 2002)

Both anxiety and Parkinson's can be viewed as offerings, challenges, qualities of Goethe's higher health (*hoehere Gesundheit*) to be tamed (Boesel &Keller, 2010, p. 359). Perhaps they are *outside external phenomena* to invest "with dream meaning and feeling," whereby the inside and outside are inextricably together, yet each itself is ineluctably autonomous: an intimate autonomy. And as a unified or attuned duality I can play with, and in, both. Playing is a nonnegotiable ingredient for becoming real. And as such, playing opens to vibrations of terror, but also to the pulsation of transformation and to the throbbing of life's pulse.

Addendum: I have noted that dreams often offer us cryptic images *inside*, reflecting our *outside* lives. Once we have *played* with them, witnessed and digested salient content material and movement, dreams can also offer guidance. I have played especially with one dream during this part of the voyage, with a dream whose guidance remains obscure, yet whose conscious accompaniment releases any frozen quality of ice. I have felt the ice melting. And the mirror...the mirror is becoming more and more like Alice's mirror…a reflection of the inside and the outside, and at the same time, when oppositional white and black cats lead Alice to the mirror, it laughs and opens. It is an entrance to another world, to a secret garden (Hodgson Burnett, 1949) to a world where Alice experiences a dreamlike real-(ality), where the Red Queen in Alice's looking glass believes six impossible things before breakfast, and where Alice's crippled cousin, Colon, regains his health (Carroll, 1865/2009). I can sense tremors of hope and can envision Aphrodite's interest, her disposition to offer a *love to me*. Every time I play with these specific dream contents, I can envision—like Galatea's experience—becoming real.

Shortly before Anna left this time, I was offered this guidance dream, which I will register as an experience of being carried by a wave to gently sway us to the next part of the voyage. My wonder, awe, and trembling increase with the fiery and compelling dynamism of this process.

I, as observer, see four newborn kittens, all with strawberry-blonde striped fur. Each kitten is, nonetheless, singularly different. One kitten—positioned on the left side of the presenting picture—is talking. I note his perfect linguistic ability, his eloquence. A second kitten—situated more to the right—has open eyes, but they are blank. Frightening. A gray color, round. A third kitten—lower right—is physically diminutive and delicate. She is in danger. The fourth kitten—center right—is normal, both psychically and physically. I just cut myself a piece of upside-down gingerbread. It tastes fantastic! The third kitten, the delicate one, meows and says: "May I have a taste?"

Molt 10: The disunion

It's no longer a dualistic Old Testament contest like between Ahab and the whale, nor is it an "or" between red or white, or between the on or off phases of Parkinson's disease. It is not the fate that the poet claims: "finding oneself opposite/and only that and always opposite." Rather, it slowly becomes more of a "pure space into which flowers endlessly bloom" and "fountains run into eternity" (Rilke, 1992) [71]

---

[71] The relevant portion of "The Eighth Elegy" is italicized and located in Appendix A-12.

When I wake up at night and cannot get up, when I lie in bed waiting for a connection between my wanting to get up and my body's marble Galatea-immobility, when I recognize that there is no communication between the two, I take 50 mg of dopamine and I breathe. Up until now, I've viewed the breath as a kind of umbilical cord between these two venues; up until now the breath was something I made use of; up until now it was part of the "world/ and never Nowhere…" (Rilke, 1992). Instead of a space of nothingness to dare to enter, there was a solidified distance, which my breath was employed to disperse. An act, a *doing*, instead of a *being*. And, as usual, when I *do*—I am either successful or I fail. There was no *nothing* or never *nowhere*, an autonomous entity, a space I do not have to enter and *do*, a space that could also grant a chance to "endlessly bloom" and "run into Eternity."

Instead of being concerned exclusively with the act of breathing, I now know the noun *breath*. I know breath as a space, as a constituted vacuum of nothingness where the world and eternity meet. And there I hover. And I gradually settle into a kind of circulatory rhythm. And I am curious. And I am faintly fearful. I feel now, not so much a war of opposites, but rather, a circular vibrating continuum of change, a firming of something that feels like a newly sculptured central core. I recall Jung's reference to a "bilateral activity of the point in the centre" that represents an emotional realization of opposites, and this realization gradually leads, or should lead, to their equilibrium. … This vacillating between the opposites and being tossed back and forth means contained *in* the opposites. They become a vessel in which what was previously now one thing and now another floats vibrating, so that the painful suspension between opposites gradually changes into the bilateral activity of the point in the centre. (Jung, 1984, Bd. 14/1, para. 290)[72]

---

[72] Bd. 14/1 para 290 "And then we begin with the so called 'freeing oneself' from the opposites, known as the nirdvanda in Indian philosophy. This is actually a psychological process rather than a philosophical one." Bd. 14/I para 290, pp. 256-257 (Danach kuendigt sich die sogenannte 'Befreiung von den Gegensaetzen, das nirdvanda der indischen Philosophen, an, was ja nicht eigentliche eine philosphische, sondern vielmehr eine psychologische Entwicklung ist….).

Parkinson's asserts its limiting, undefined, yet paradoxically clear borders of on and off, but yet in this new third space, the ossified opposites are becoming increasingly more liquid. Alchemically, they seem to be *dissolving themselves in their own water; they* learn then to become *decently unconscious* (Edinger, 1995, p 86). These once upon a time dualistic, conflicting opposites gradually learn a new dance of difference and sameness: a coalition of movement, vibration, rhythm of confederation and contradiction—an intimate autonomy. The center point hosting all this activity is the *chi*, the circulating life force, in my lower abdomen. The gingerbread is upside-down yet intuits now a new space, an interstice of savory scent between the pears and cake. Is there such a thing as a gingerbread soul? I feel faint, lightheaded, twirled, unfurled. Fearful. Everything is going so well.

The fractured union

It all begins—the fracture, or the disunion, that is—on the day before Anna is due back. She calls up sick and reschedules her arrival for a week later than planned. When she arrives, she is still racked with

---

See also "The psychological union of the opposites is a concept, a notion, which itself expresses the evolution of the phenomenology of the process.... For when we say that the conscious and the unconscious have become one, we know that such an evolution is inconceivable. The unconscious is indeed unconscious and can therefore neither be imagined nor conceptualized" (Bd. 14 II para 207, p. 144). (Die psychologische Gegensatzvereinigung ist ein Anschauungsbegriff, der die Phaenomenologie dieses Vorganges in sich begreift...Denn, indem wir sagen, Bewusstes und Unbewusstes vereinigen sich, sprechen wir aus, dass es sich um ein unvorstellbaren Vorgang handelt. Das Unbewusste ist naemlich unbewusst und kann daher weder erfasst noch vorgestellt werden.)

See also "This circular movement generates the moral connotations of all the dark and light forces of human nature, and with that includes all possible psychological opposites no matter what kind they might be. This means getting to know yourself through birthing yourself, through self evolution" (Bd. 13, para. 38, p. 34). (Die Kreisbewegung hat demnach auch die moralische Bedeutung aller hellen und dunkeln Kraefte menschlicher Natur, und damit aller psychologischen Gegensaetzte, welcher Art sie auch sein moegen. Das bedeutet nichts anderes als Selbsterkenntnis durch Selbstbebruetung. See also Bd 13, para. 104.

coughs, which, with a loud volume and staccato rhythm, signals for me an unequivocal rupture of her good-enough mothering. I feel our roles are beginning to become transposed. Our carefully woven relationship of my dependency and Anna's nurture is suddenly and abruptly torn asunder. No longer is she omnipotent; no longer can I count on her unfailing boundless accessibility; no longer does the space between Anna and me feel round, contained, cuddly, soft, and safe.

We have become a separate two; we are no more a two-in-a-one of an intimate autonomy. We have become an intersubjective relationship: We are in a space now with a pattern for two, each demanding disconnected blueprints etching out respective boundaries of give and take. Separate boundaries instead of autonomous liquid borders; we have become a disunion. And for this meeting we have comparatively such a short space of time: a period of only three and a half weeks to become acquainted with and to adjust to this new rhythm. Or to rechoreograph the dance.

I feel submerged. I have lost my breath.

The white cat

A dream: I am living with a white cat: We eat together, we sleep together, we play together. Not suddenly—but rather slowly, adagio, as "written" music, as if it is fate, around a corner and into our house we watch a flash flood surge toward us. Three times the obtrusive water bursts in on us and then recedes. The fourth time my white cat gets up and simply walks into the water as it begins to recede. As if she were going to play with the waves, or wash herself, or…or as if she simply knows that it is time.

Upon awaking I know I am to follow.

This part of the voyage seems to be about the usual inter-personal/intrapsychic dance of closeness and of distance; it is about being opened, about yielding, about sacrificing defenses, repetitive compulsive structures. It's not only about giving up. Even though there are those moments. It's about giving in.

Up and *in* could be opposites in this context, they could get stuck in a fate of "being opposite and nothing more than opposite and always that"[73]...or they could begin playing...or dancing ...they could toss each other *upside and down* like the dough and the pears of the gingerbread, a dynamic at least potentially sparking further movement. Oppositional energies are an invitation to dance with an 'Other,' to play, to find a rhythm, an attunement where a twirling swirls and activates a center, where the opposites of vertical and horizontal cross and then nest. And something new is birthed. They can become still in a place of horizontal verticality, where the opposites of red and white first struggle and surge against each other before igniting perhaps a fire (red) in the water (white), where the shifts between the ons and the offs of Parkinson's transmute to slides and then perhaps glide into a "pure space where flowers endlessly bloom." And within this alchemical "absolute unity of the unity and the difference" something new can be spawned (Giegerich, 1995, p. 120). Once an old pattern can be un-locked, a new constellation can emanate from the vibrating *chi* energy inhabiting the bilateral point in the center.

Or the opposites can stagnate, secure a disunion. It is then an empty space, rather than a *fecund nothingness*. It becomes Rilke's conviction of fate to be *opposite and nothing more than opposite and always that*.

The structure of Anna's and my relationship has to be redesigned. Following "the rupture," the new ingredients demand the creation of a new gestalt, both qualitatively and quantitatively. Our newly transmuted third space (that is not a third *space)* includes—the painter appreciates—"the unity of movement...the first thing to seize upon... is the direction of your main movement, the sweep of the whole thing as a unit.... For long I have been trying to get these movements of the parts," the artist explained. "Now I see there is only one movement. It sways and ripples...but it is only one movement sweeping out into space but always keeping going." (Shadbolt, 1987, p. 175) My whole

---

[73] German translation: "gegenueber sein/und nichts als das und immer gegenueber..."

body seems to be one "swaying and rippling" movement or one un-movement. Anna is confused. Our relationship is in a state of upheaval. What is our "one movement"?

At first, the old parts and patterns refuse to dislodge. Then this happens: I begin to become increasingly irritated with Anna's incessant coughing. It steals the spotlight from me. I—my body—begin(s) to become stuck in the off parts. In this case, my infant omnipotence sparks its perpetual projected opposite of devaluation, and I began to spin into a state of rigid personal and projected negativity. Admitted, there are fiercely difficult moments for me, moments again of frozen knowings, such as "there is no point in trying anymore," the oppositional space of success or of failure, the space where there is no playing, no sliding into a circular dance of trying and then letting it be, back and forth and forth and back. And I feel a seething rage at Anna and at Parkinson's and at their interminable commanding presence in my life. And I feel justified and right. And compelling also is a kind of addictive energy I feel, a powerful need to return home, to my on and off oppositional place, to a place of familiarity, to a place known, to my accustomed position of ego control. I know this need: It is clinically a repetition compulsion. But at least there, there hovers no doubt.

Following a couple of these affect-laden hysterical dramas, Anna reminds me that I am sabotaging her personally as well as also our mutual process, that with my narcissistic and destructive Snow Queen behavior, my "freezing," I am being seduced by Thanatos, the empty pure white part of the Freudian repetition compulsion, and am not allowing its opposite movement, the red of Eros, of change, of growth, any room whatsoever.[74] She reminds me of a story I used to tell, which

---

[74] Freud introduced this notion in chapters 3 and 4 of Beyond the Pleasure Principle (1920), making it one of the new foundations of his theory. He considered the repetition compulsion as a largely dominant "universal attitude of organic life in general." Unconscious instincts are also subject to this law. In his later works, Freud emphasized the destructiveness of the repetition compulsion. He viewed the destructive instinct as a death instinct (Thanatos) and its opposite, the life instinct, he called Eros. For me, Freud's repetition compulsion is one of his most important discoveries, i.e., a realization of patterns unconsciously and compulsively repeating themselves.

hints at her frustration at my slow ability to follow the white cat, to give in, to accept our new unfamiliar rhythm. Instead, Anna points out, I am perpetuating the oppositional immobility while stonewalling any unity of movement. Anna recalls this anecdote:

The narcissist

Along with other prominent people in Frankfurt society, a famous actor was invited to a formal dinner. It is a known custom in Germany that such a dinner enjoys the ritual that the man undertakes the entertainment of the woman sitting to his right. Our actor is pleased to relate one story after another about himself to the attractive woman seated next to him.

The evening drags on until after the dessert, and just as the coffee is being served, our actor looks at the woman (really for the first time), and politely asks, "Mein Gott! I've been talking about myself all the evening. Let's talk about you for a change: What do you think of my latest film?"

Such a person is positioned "opposite/and nothing more than opposite and always that." The distance our actor keeps from his companion has such a range that the other—if seen at all—is perceived as a separate and foreign part; she is seen perhaps at the most "through a glass darkly." There is no real communication, no dialogue between two. I think about the loneliness of the eagle and of our little king wren.

I get it. The humor of this forgotten story, however, seems to remain stuck in my throat.

Anna is right. I am too distanced from her. I have lost her. I have lost our process. I have lost our third space and its playful attempts to attain an autopoietical oppositional attunement. The humming of our fugue of autonomy and unity, even the screams of our deserted relating pattern of intimate autonomy, a structure endemic in the third space, have become empty notes of mute echoes.

But what about Anna? A disunion is a break of twos. What has been her part, her need to distance? What is her contribution to the disunion?

Part Three

Molt 9: The Dragonfly

I feel an impulse to digress slightly and to relate at this point how the dragonfly and I met.

My relationship with the dragonfly begins in 2009 with my confrontation once again with the question: What is reality? To recapitulate: My feeling real does not come from rational, logical, ordered thinking, but rather during the minutes or seconds or hours of creativity, spontaneity, the substance of the third space of play. I do not get stuck in the credulity of others, but rather I live on a causality line stretching its length with every moment spurred by energies emanating from want (narcissism), fear of losing control (schizoid splitting), or the chaos of not knowing, and feelings of meaninglessness (depression), among other clinically captured archetypes. If my only other choice is to fall *victim* to Freud's pleasure principle by not living in the reality space, then I am condemned to potential *insanity*, and I am driven by Freud's ensuing revisionary elaboration of the pleasure principle in 1920—by Thanatos, the death instinct, which lures me back to my original state of living in the world "which, though based on *play*, does not involve a betrayal of the self in compliance and imitation."

It all begins like this:

One early morning bathed in the pink rays of early sunshine and the mists of light rain, I enter my practice to discover a light-blue *living flash of light*, a seemingly young, small dragonfly. How can it be here? The thought dances in my head with its sense of rational arrogance. The doors and windows are shut! I want to continue writing my book!

The sadness, the helplessness of being imprisoned in this room, anxiety when I appear...all this I sense that the dragonfly feels. As I watch this tiny blue insect, I am struck by the ephemeral yet incandescent quality of its wings, but also by the strength, the unswerving, linear arrow-straight in the tail. This oppositional two-in-one, fragile, elfinlike being. I open a window, the dragonfly flies away with darting missilelike speed. I remain imprisoned in my room and in the Parkinsonian incarceration. Pierced with pinpricks of envy, I burst into tears.

The summer of the dragonfly continues. Weird, unusual, fascinating. Real. Encounters with my spirit animal.

A couple of weeks later, a person dear to me brings me a black dragonfly, dead, but still in perfect form, like an intricately carved ebony sculpture. A few weeks after that, on my black bedroom carpet where I do yoga exercises before going to bed, another dragonfly lies, black also, defying the dust of death, she, too, a piece of sculptured suspension. At the end of the summer, sometime in August, at the end of a walk, my husband and I stopped at a picnic table to rest. This time she was a small, red dragonfly. She flies up to me, stops, hovers right in front of my eyes, as if to say: "Get on with it, Meredith!"[75]

After this summer's experience with these weirdly invasive dragonflies, I feel an intimacy, a closeness with the dragonfly that eventually leads me to an astonished moment of comprehension: This must be how one encounters a spirit animal. Nothing else makes any sense. Since that time, the dragonfly has become part of my innermost core.

My dance with the dragonfly: Peering into the looking glass

For me, much of the dragonfly's experience during its transmutation seems to reflect so often my own development. Or my development seems to mirror the dragonfly's transmutation. Perhaps one of a spirit animal's tasks is to provide a looking glass that *holds* until its scaffolding function becomes interiorized, until it becomes a core part of me. And perhaps this is my function for my dragonfly.

The dragonfly and me

The first task of the dragonfly is to hatch; for some in cooler climates, the egg takes longer to break. Once out of the egg, the dragonfly can

---

[75] I will be describing this 2009 summer of the dragonfly, at times quoting directly from my article published in Psychological Perspectives, Vol. 52, Issue 1, pp. 37-54.

move, and life (and potential trauma) begins: *Thrashing and flipping*, it must find water immediately or it dies within seconds. In the water, the dragonfly becomes more mobile. It commences its existence as a predator. The first molt (which from a scientist's perspective—and from ours—is the last molt) is the metamorphosis from a prolarva to a nymph, or aquatic larva. (Perhaps one could *see* a tiny ego being formed; perhaps due to the water experience or the experience of an encounter with the unconscious, ego layers become evident in the rapacious need to eat and the inevitable consequential "gift" of the feces. (I remember reading Freud's theory about the child and his feces. The infant regards its feces as part of its own body; feces represent an infant's first present to the environment. By producing feces, he can express his active compliance, and by withholding them, he expresses his disobedience).

Dragonflies are carnivorous in all larva stages and as adults. Their digestive system is more intricate and yet similar to other insects. The basic body plan of the dragonfly remains the same until the nymph enters the adult stage, but an adaptation special to the dragonfly is the larva's prevention of fecal material from contaminating the rectal cavity and fouling the oxygen exchange surfaces. As food passes through the intestinal tract and becomes digested, it is encased in a membrane derived from the gut surface and formed into a pellet. This pellet is ejected, sometimes quite forcefully, from the rectum and away from the larva.

The anal opening to the rectum is through the 10th abdominal segment and is constricted. When the dragonfly larva wants to move quickly or suspend itself in the water, it can, by contracting the abdomen, force water from the rectum through the anal opening and jet propel itself through the water, rather like a squid or an octopus. Conversely, when the larva attacks prey, a constricting mechanism seals the opening of the rectum and prevents the release of a jet of water. Otherwise, the larva would launch itself through the water at a time when it needs stealth and a steady aim to capture its meal. Jet propulsion is a special feature of the dragonfly larva. (Stool retention or constipation is a typical symptom of Parkinson's disease. Even though I have experienced little increased ability to concentrate or focus due to constipation, and—for that matter—I've not been able to jet-stream myself from one place to another, my relationship with feces has increased in intensity and the recent shift from constipation to regular daily stools has reflected yet another kinship with the dragonfly. I feel more with my body instead of being caught in a dualistic power battle between my will and my body. Perhaps I could now even jet stream a "pellet" and shoot up from the toilet. Or I could hold a bowel movement and be curious if my conscious concentration increases. And the stool does feel like a gift to me and to the relationship between Parkinson's and me, perhaps in the sense of a transitional object. This more regular stool has contributed to my emergence into the adult stage.)

Even though the basic structure and form of the dragonfly larva does not change, what redesigns is the repetitive molting, or shedding, of an "exoskeleton." A scaffoldlike structure, a snakelike skin, is shed.

Because insects have their exoskeleton on the outside of their bodies, they cannot grow the way humans do. Their exoskeleton stretches only so far, so if they need to get any bigger, they need a bigger exoskeleton. So, they grow a new, bigger one under the smaller one. This exoskeleton is so soft and flexible that the whole thing can fit underneath. Then the old exoskeleton is shed to allow the new one. For the dragonfly, this process takes place 10 to 15 times, the average being 12 molts. The dragonfly seems to know when this transmutation is to take place.

When an insect molts, it breaks out and stretches out by inhaling a lot of air and pushing fluids around inside its body. When it's fully expanded, the smaller, older exoskeleton breaks open, and the new, larger exoskeleton hardens. Each molting process precipitates the next. At some point, an insect undergoes a final molt and become an adult. Once an insect is an adult, it no longer molts. This means that insects only molt when they are preadults, or immatures.

(It must be something like a baby shedding an exoskeleton the moment it can hold its head erect. We also hold a basic form and structure throughout life. But unlike the dragonfly, our growth does not include the exoskeleton as scaffold to then be shed. Rather, our repetition compulsions can reflect the containing scaffolds, but intrapsychically. When we can begin to gradually shed our defensive, protective compulsions, we are able to contain forces such as anxiety and can become more and more exposed, less protected, more vulnerable. And more independent. This process, this molting, can gently unfold into an intimate autonomy.)

The dragonfly is unable to grow unless it sheds the old exoskeleton and grows a new one. Up to 15 exoskeletons are shed, 12 being the most common. The duration of this molting can be six months or longer. The dragonfly's life as a larva can last from two to six years. (It takes much longer to shed a repetition compulsion.) This molting period is a critical time in the life of the dragonfly, a time during which it is defenseless against predators and bad weather. (Letting go of old patterns feels like daring to be naked, daring to feel these old patterns, daring to get close enough to them to let them go. In order to *touch* these old patterns, in order to feel these patterns, regression is more often than not the *via regia*: *Thrashing and flipping* to try to avoid a return to *earlier waters* could suggest the terror of regression's possible exposure to the pain of an early trauma.)

No matter how many molts the larva makes, there is no difficulty in determining which one is the last one, after which the adult can emerge. The dragonfly ceases feeding and looks for a safe place outside of water. When one is found, its legs stiffen and lock to the surface. Then emergence begins. The skin of the larva along the top of the thorax begins to split; the back of the head capsule may also break open. The adult pushes up and out of the skin, sometimes falling backward toward the water. The abdomen remains encased in the larval skin, however, and can be an anchor allowing the process to continue. As the adult legs pull free, the empty skin hardens, and the legs act as clamps to hold the emerging dragonfly in place. The adult flops forward, and its legs help pull the abdomen from the skin. At this point, the wings are tiny, and the body is soft and shiny. But then the body begins to contract, and hemolymph is pumped into the wing veins, which are as pliable and delicate as thin tissue. The wings expand as the hemolymph fills the veins. Slowly they inflate, still translucent as opposed to transparent. Once the wings are full-size, the veins and vessels begin to harden. Patience is required for this phase. The dragonfly has to be dry to fly.

(I currently feel the need to break out of my former skin, to take off and to dare to live. I've experienced my legs "attaching," I've experienced my skin as delicate and pliable as thin tissue; for example, I've felt invaded, I've felt like the exposure burns, and I've felt myself "flopping backward into the water" again and again. Interspersed, I've known the feeling of a contracting body and expanding wings lending me a strength and presence hitherto unknown. But the patience required demands perhaps a meditative orientation and positioning.)

In flight, the legs compose a basket underneath the dragonfly's body while the wings unfold. Indispensable to life's plan, hauntingly intricate in design, and uniquely structured and constructed to birth, to enhance life's time on earth, the wings of the dragonfly are un-paralleled in their unity of objective beauty and subjective functionality. The speed of the dragonfly, its ability to stop and to take off, its paradoxical pattern to hover and to dart, its life juices of blood and oxygen, as well its beauty of colors and grace…all this is in the hermetic wings of the dragonfly: a functional inner scaffold of blood and of breath ensuring life while simultaneously, "seen through the lens of the artist, the mitochondrial veins chisel geometric patterns and transform the wings into ancient tiny mirrors…the wings of the dragonfly appear to be translucent, evanescent sheets of shimmering mica." (Oenning-Hodgson, 2009, pp. 50-51)

The beauty and apparent fragility of the dragonfly often belies her physical strength and versatility. Like a dancer or an athlete, she appears to be unencumbered by the elemental dualities of earth and air. Developmentally, the dragonfly begins as a water nymph and matures to a winged reproductive adult, incarnating a purposeful mixture of otherwise unrelated elements. Reflecting this biological *third*, the dragonfly appears delicate, innocent, and beautiful while assumedly harboring hidden, secret, potential evil. In German, the word for the dragonfly is *Teufelsnadel*, meaning "the Devil's needle."[76] (Perhaps my emergence could be accelerated if I would begin consciously to use my *Teufelsnadel* instead of fearing it as a "hidden, secret potential evil." Thinking of Jung's notion that the "shadow is the backbone of the ego," perhaps Parkinson's as my shadow, which "violently interrupted my life," *is* a gift of the gods!)

Dreams

Almost immediately following this moment of recognition and acknowledgment, I have three important dreams, which I want to relate in short form. Each seems to reach back to and gather a thread from the "four kittens dream": Each dream ignites interconnection between the unconscious and the conscious, rendering them into a one unified "movement sweeping out into space." (Shadbolt, p. 1987, 175) At the same time, each dream maintains its own respective autonomy, each "seize(s) upon the direction of the main movement: a kind of recollection of scattered units or sparks of light into an ordered, centered unity." (von Franz, 1980, p. 169)[77] I want to reconnect with this key dream at the end of Molt 11 and then summarize these subsequent dreams occurring later:

(In the four kittens dream, I, as observer, see four newborn kittens, all with strawberry-blonde striped fur. Each kitten is singularly different. One kitten—positioned on the left side of the presenting picture—is talking. I note his perfect linguistic ability, his eloquence. A second kitten—situated more to the right—has open eyes, but they are blank. Frightening. A gray color, round. A third kitten—lower right—is

---

[76] Most of the facts regarding the dragonfly are taken from F. L. Mitchell & J. L. Lasswell (2005).

[77] Recall the dream!

physically diminutive and delicate. She is in danger. The fourth kitten—center right—is normal, both psychically and physically.)

Dream One:

During this part of the voyage, I am taken out of water and am put on land. Symbolically, I am not in the unconscious anymore, not anymore in water but on the earth, in a more conscious place. I am excavating large sections of land in search of my home, searching for a place familiar and known to me. I can hear the eloquent kitten lecturing on some ancient city hidden under the earth somewhere in this area. The diction, the grammar, the syntax—the structural—the kitten-lecturer has it down perfectly. And I as a listener? I feel exchangeable. The eloquent kitten could have been lecturing to (at) anyone. Any feeling connection to this first kitten is missing.

Dream Two:

In the next dream, my sister and I arrive at the border of the United States with a van full of children to be adopted. One is a young boy from India. I am holding him in such a way that only one of his eyes is visible. But this single eye suddenly looks at me. Without blinking, the eye holds its penetrating gaze. This eye is perfectly round, no eyelashes, gray, and unusual in its concentrated intensity, in its depth and its strength. Then, this East Indian boy gradually begins to grow; he grows and grows and grows…until he is about nine years of age. The moment in the dream that remains with me is our three eyes meeting: my two eyes and his one eye.

I remember the blind cat in my former dream and recall Tiresias, the blind seer in Homer's *Odyssey* and in T. S. Eliot's *Wasteland*. He or she views as "in a mirror dimly." (I Corinthians 13:12) He, who once was a woman, sees from all sides. In both stories, he/she sees with an inner eye of recognition, which mediates a different view of ourselves than does the ego. Only through this eye can a human being really see himself. It is as if an *inner eye* watches us; one's eyes are opened. Von Franz describes the eye in a dream as a "divine eye, which, so to speak, looks at us from within and in whose seeing lies the only nonsubjectively colored source of knowledge." (von Franz, 1980, p. 166; see also Giegerich, 2012, p. 125)[78]

I feel seen by the blind cat. Not seen like the woman in the narcissist story, but really seen and perceived. But perceived by a force foreign to me, from whose wellspring I feel imbued with a new kind of confidence and strength. It feels as if an accompanying presence, a self-evolving entity is going to be *in me* throughout eternity, a presence that would never abandon me, a presence akin to the soul of the early depth analyst—if not the first: Heraclitus. He views soul as truth, so deep "you could not find the ends of the soul though you travelled every way, so deep is its logos." (Hillman, 1979, p. 25) Truth reigns at a depth akin to *knowing* (*kennen*).

The dragonfly...my spirit animal. ... Suddenly, I remember reading specifically about its strange eyes: How do dragonflies survive while even dinosaurs became extinct? Perhaps they see more. The eyes of the dragonfly are like giant kaleidoscopes. Lenses of varied sizes, hues, and shapes, each faces a different direction. Each lens holds a different image. The dragonfly's brain gathers scattered and varied information, and like the pieces of a kaleidoscope after being shaken, one picture is formed and settles. Dragonflies see far more than any other insect; they seem to be able to see even beyond, for they know exactly when to cease to feed several days before they leave the water and shed their last exoskeleton to emerge as an adult. Their eyes seem to perceive knowledge of a nonsubjective nature. It sometimes feels like dragonfly eyes have claimed a space behind my eyes. I can now *see* through their eyes—or the dragonfly looks through my eyes. Or some other entity looks through our eyes, first at us, and then out into the world. Whenever it chooses to do so.

---

[78] Meister Eckhart: "The soul is like a ball of fire or a fire eye. Only through this eye can a human being really see himself and partake of the nature of God, who himself is all eye." "The eye through which I see God is the same eye through which God sees me; my eye and God's eye are one eye, one seeing, one knowing, one love." See also Giegerich: "The soul makes itself: it becomes true to itself—even if only through humans...a prayer is only a true prayer if it is already God who through one's human praying is speaking the prayer to God, in other words, NOT the human person per se—not the ego."

Dream Three:

The third dream is a kind of vision in that seminal space between sleeping and being awake: My infant me (the diminutive, delicate kitten) and I are outside in a space like the Red Rock Theater outside Denver, Colorado, where I was born. Suddenly, a large lion emerges from behind one of the rocks. My first reaction is one of fear and of panic, but that yields quickly to awe and to curiosity. For one lion follows after another until there is a ring of lions around us. When the circle is complete, when an uroboros form emerges and for a moment remains still, then a kind of dance begins: The lions slowly transform to humans and then back to lions and then back to humans ad infinitum. These transformations slide. They seem to be in a continual process of birthing themselves (Bebruetung, autopoiesis). It is a symphony of many different notes, a dance of different rhythms, sounds resounding and rebounding from rock to rock in one single sweep, swaying and rippling, vibrating echoes in and out of the mountains and up into the heavens.

The delicate kitten just stands and watches. I can hear in the distance and I recognize the haunting chords of Pergolesi's Stabat Mater (1736) ("The Sorrowful Mother Stands"), my favorite among the many musical renditions of this 13th-century poem.

There remains one significant moment to chronicle in this part of the voyage: the new experience of my body being one and many, a conflation, a *unified multiplicity*, a somatic fugue. My head, the upper part of my body, my legs—each contributing to a tone resounding, pulsating from a single center. Once again, a third space reveals a harbored paradoxical fugue of fluid solidity.

The painter with the canvas, the sculptor with the block of marble, the composer with the blank score...an artist has a vision, which is not known until seen on canvas, or which reveals itself as the marble assumes form, or the composer's notes on the lined score become music. An artist is someone who goes beyond rendering a likeness to release something new or hidden. The artist sees beyond herself, beyond the other: the canvas, the marble, the musical score. She sees the one movement. The painter, Emily Carr, describes the process:

"When I paint a tree, I sit in front of the tree. And then I wait until I see God in the tree. I remain sitting. I wait until I see God in me. Only then do I paint." (Shadbolt, 1987, pp. 195-196) She sees the one movement in herself, in the tree, and in God. Then she paints.

Like a good-enough mother, who can give of herself without losing herself, who can simultaneously be sufficiently self-assertive, who can likewise in a child *release something new or hidden*, the artist knows a space of soul, of comprehending a space where distance and closeness are "now one thing, now another...an emotional realization of opposites," a space undulating rhythmically, where the child is contained and simultaneously free to birth itself (*Bebruetung*). Both the artist and the mother know the one true dance of creativity: "the direction of (the) main movement, the sweep of the whole thing as a unit...one movement. It sways and ripples...but it is only one movement sweeping out into space but always keeping going." (Shadbolt, 1987, pp. 195-196) One movement yet paradoxically activated by the bilateral energies of confederation and contradiction, the "bilateral activity of the point in the centre." (Jung, 1982, Bd. 13, para. 104; *1984,* Bd. 14)[79] A crystal reflecting the structures and the hues of an intimate autonomy.

The fracture...the disunion, is it part of a birth process? Or is the rupture a regressive but at least a semiconscious tearing, disclosing a dynamic pregnant challenge to the poet's conviction of the irrefutable fate *to be opposite/and nothing more than opposite and always that*? Does Emily Carr's intimate autonomy with the tree and with God and with herself refute this?

In a month Anna returns from Frankfurt for our next meeting. When she leaves here, her cough is gone. Toward the end of her stay, after her health becomes stabilized, we both catch ourselves slipping into our old roles: she as the good-enough mother and I as the infant. It is different from before, however, because we would both slide into these former identifications and then out...in and out and out and in.

---

[79] "The dragon slays itself, weds itself, and impregnates itself."

And then often into a third space, a new space. An echo of the rhythm of the lions?

In fairy tales there are often three tasks to accomplish before the prince or princess is won. Regarding the imminent next section of the voyage, once again curiosity reigns, even while fear sneaks in. And the fourth kitten, the "normal," more adapted kitten, is waiting to leave the water and return to land. Perhaps she has already accomplished her three tasks…perhaps she is going to study us…perhaps she is a mirror of my body experience of *one and many*. … Perhaps she is part of me because she is in my dream and yet will behave even more autonomously than Goethe's Mephistopheles, when the author begins once again to finish his drama. Goethe feels terror when he considers returning to *Faust* and continuing his 60-year "journey" with the Devil (Trunz, 1996, p. 431).[80]

In view of the fact that Mephistopheles seems to take off on his own, when he does return to his writing, Goethe finds himself paralyzed with fear when dealing with his self-conjured antihero. Mephisto's autonomy scares Goethe so much that he cannot continue writing *Faust* without his friend and colleague, Friedrich Schiller's presence. He has to be physically with Schiller, who has to then mirror, who has to confirm, indeed, to *real-alize* what Goethe writes.[81]

---

[80] On the 6th of April 1800, Goethe wrote Schiller: Der Teufel, den ich beschwoere, gebaerdet sich sehr wunderlich. (Author's translation: The devil, whom I myself conjure, is behaving quite strangely.)

[81] Clinically, Schiller fills the chasm that remains a Nothingness, empty and without even the sound of a hiss for the brilliant and creative German author. Due to his traumatic birth, his lack of good-enough mothering, Goethe remains perhaps unable to cope with the intimacy of a relationship. The vertical— rather than the horizontal—split leaves the author terrified of being alone. The pulsating beat of the repetition compulsion's structure catches Goethe continually in its net. The pressure of this space of the Mothers—described so poignantly in Faust II (lines 6230-6290), where Faust must learn to be with Emptiness [my translation]: Learn 'Emptiness, teach Nothingness' (Das Leere lernen, Leere lehren, line 6232). The space of the Mothers sets the stage for his repetitive falling in love, his inability to enter such an intimacy, and then leave the relationship—or to unconsciously or consciously use this fiery energy of spurned love and its residual terrifying threat of the emptiness of Nothingness, to compulsively fill it with his writing.

Perhaps my fourth kitten will usher me into realms I don't want to enter. Perhaps my "normal" fourth kitten—like the white whale in Melville's *Moby Dick*—will unveil Evil, and I will engage in a mirrored memory of Ahab's solipsistic, red "fiery hunt." (Melville, 1847/1967, pp. 717-718)[82] Or perhaps when Anna is here, her presence will be able to contain me during an ontological shift. Perhaps I can shed a false self and step into my own reality. Or perhaps...

Molt 8: The Pitbull and the kitten: a two-in-one movement

Perhaps...I have noted at the end of Molt 9. These three dots mean something like "to be continued." It could be that the dots are compelling in that they are there, and they are not there. The three dots express nothing, and at the same time they evoke a kind of spirit of inquiry about something through their having expressed nothing.

And it concerns the last of the four kittens, the kitten who is "normal and adapted," the kitten who seems to be the least complicated. What is it about this fourth kitten? Is she the only one of the four who can hold the tension of an intimate autonomy with the white whale? Where is this kitten going to take us? The three dots leave it open. This openness can kindle curiosity. It can also create a vacuum, a space of empty nothingness, which can evoke fear. Or it can at times invoke a dance between fear and curiosity, a relating pattern instead of the more common defensive fight/flight or freeze reaction.

Like the sudden dart of the dragonfly when it launches flight in a different direction, a dream in this part of our anaclitic odyssey opens and releases a hitherto relatively unfamiliar energy. This nighttime adventure seems to demand the shedding of a repetition compulsive structure, which frees an energy or an entity latently held at a detached

---

[82] "Ahab had cherished a wild vindictiveness against the whale, all the more fell for that in his frantic morbidness he at last came to identify with him, not only his bodily woes, but all his intellectual and spiritual exasperations...all evil, to crazy Ahab, were visibly personified, and made practically assailable in Moby Dick."

distance by unconscious splitting. It is the last dream I have before Anna returns to Germany, a dream reminiscent of Ahab's rage at the white whale, a dream escalating and supplementing the kitten dream, a dream that concentrates specifically on the one kitten not yet dealt with, the fourth kitten:

The pitbull

I own a puppy. It grows up quickly and soon is as large as a small pony. The face, the fierce face, is highlighted in my dream: It is enlarged; it takes up the complete dream space. It is a face reflecting rage, seething violence, a snarling need to confront and to attack. The face is chillingly terrorizing. There is only one person able to relate with this dog: I have the task—and the ability—only I—to calm this pitbull, to relate with him, to curtail any imminent threat to an "Other."

And this is the transformed, transmogrified normal, adapted, cuddly, strawberry-blonde kitten? What has happened in these few weeks to summon up the pitbull?

"And what rough beast, its hour come around at last...Can the centre hold" (Yeats, 1919)?[83]

Perhaps the oppositional qualities of the fourth kitten and the pitbull mirror the experience of my body being one and many. Does every body have at least two and probably more energies? The kitten and the pitbull are two, but are they also one? In me? Perhaps with the appearance of the pitbull, my kitten is going to unveil a part of herself that can be evil. But this kitten is the more adapted, the more normal one! Is evil normal, is evil adapted, attuned to me and to my surroundings? Is evil perhaps—as the black poodle hatching the Devil in *Faust* divulges—"I am part of that energy which consistently wants to do Evil/ And consistently ends up doing Good?" (*Faust*, 1806/1992, line 1335) Could that energy be the kitten and the pitbull playing

---

[83] The full text of Yeat's poem "The Second Coming" is located in Appendix A-8.

together: the kitten representing the good, the pitbull, evil? Could the kitten and the pitbull be a two in the one of an intimate autonomy? Could this reflect an entity—or entities—in Anna—or for that matter also in me…and assumedly in everybody—that many of us are unaware of?

In my body the oppositional energetic directions between my kitten and my pitbull could feel like a kind of crucifixion were they to remain static oppositional forces, each pulling in the other direction. Or if further disassociated, they can be so far away from each other in a vertical split that there is not even a faint echo of a heartbeat to be interchanged. Such a split often makes itself known somatically. Like Parkinson's disease.

The horizontal split does not routinely create such a distance between the opposites—or the twos. But with the vertical split there are physical tones to be heard and felt in the empty space between. It can feel like being held in a paralysis by Parkinsonian clamps, screws tightened at different intervals—unfortunately, a familiar experience. If I can be conscious enough of the potential creativity of such vibrant oppositional energies, perhaps an ossification can be broken and the freed animals (the instincts) can be encouraged to play with each other. This reconciles and unites the otherwise clashing energies, activates the bilateral point at the center, and the different parts swirl into a one, while at the same time warranting each one of the two its respective autonomy. The crucifying torment of the I-am-right-and-you-are-wrong dualism is then dissolved. The reality of an intimate autonomy begins to vibrate and then to breathe, both for the kitten and for the pitbull. Intrapsychically. And, of course, for me. And for Anna and me, interpersonally.

Contemporary brain research substantiates physical dangers emanating from stress without a porthole of play (Reynolds, 2018).[84]

---

[84] The amygdala stores memories and images and constantly watches for anything that may pose a threat. Unfortunately, we don't know what has been imprinted as a trigger for the fight-or-flight response. Let's break down how your brain processes a potential threat using the example of seeing a snake on the ground. First, the amygdala, which is constantly

THE HISS OF HOPE

If my kitten and the pitbull do not play with each other and remain ossified and static, each in its own space, the resulting tension could also feel like some symptoms of early wounding, as noted by Rene Spitz (see fn. 57). In his 1946 description of anaclitic depression, he includes depression caused by early wounding; that is, no one to lean on (no one to use) in the first six months of life. According to the latest research, resulting symptoms are sleeplessness, delayed psychomotor development, and some developed physical rigidity. These are also symptoms of Parkinson's. Could Parkinson's be a result of a psychic split due to a preverbal trauma? Could Parkinson's have forced his presence on me because unconsciously some part of me has kept the kitten and the pitbull apart from each other? Could this be a potential moment of Goethe's higher health (*hoehere Gesundheit*)? And now does Parkinson's

---

on guard, triggers the sympathetic nervous system (the emotional accelerator), and in 1/200 of a second adrenaline is released, your heart rate jumps to over 100, and you leap out of harm's way.

Next, the prefrontal cortex analyzes the type of snake to determine whether it poses a risk. If it perceives no danger, it triggers the parasympathetic nervous system, which operates as the brakes on our emotional system. This alarm system is crucial for the survival of our species. What would happen if, instead of immediately reacting, we were to stand there trying to discern the type of snake and whether it poses a risk? We'd have two fang marks on our leg long before we could determine whether we should jump out of the way. At other times anger, which is a part of the fight response, is critical if we are to survive. Reacting and then determining the potential risk significantly increases our odds of survival in the wild, but it's not always so helpful in day-to-day life.

Dynamic in nature, the amygdala is constantly adapting to its present environment. Circumstances where there is fear, pain, shame, guilt, disrespect, insults, physical danger, and/or injury are just a few of the life experiences that can be marked by the amygdala as something to watch for in order to survive. Generally our survival system tends to hum along just fine unless we experience trauma.

The amygdala, when triggered, stomps on our emotional accelerator causing us to react with either anger or by running away. The prefrontal cortex evaluates the situation to determine if there is current danger, and if none exists, it slams on our emotional brakes. This system is dependent on the prefrontal cortex being able to make sense of what is happening so it can send the other parts of the brain the appropriate signals to calm you down.

Here's where the severity of this process sets in: Severe trauma overloads the prefrontal cortex and effectively cuts the brake line to the parasympathetic nervous system, leaving us like a car with the accelerator stuck on the floorboard and no brakes. Retrieved, May 2018, from: https://www.affairrecovery.com/newsletter/founder/infidelity-betrayal-the-number-one-obstacle-to-recovery.

envision me in some kind of mediating—and attuning—role also between the kitten and the pitbull? They are so different from each other. Perhaps as mediator, my greatest task is to shepherd them into a mutual leaning on each other. Leaning on Anna, using Anna, has been one of the most difficult patterns for me to play with in our anaclitic therapy. I can appreciate Spitz's according the word *preeminence* when discussing his *anaclitic depression*. The inability to *lean*—or to use—would hinder the formation of an intimate autonomy. This inability incarnates in a rigid defense against even the tiniest spark of intimacy, against even a moment of play.

Fractals

In the 1960s and 1970s, a French mathematician, Benoit Mandelbrot, invented a mathematical language to deal with such related yet different aspects of nature (in our case, of life): He called it a "language to speak of clouds." (Mandelbrot, quoted in Capra, 1996, p. 138) This language describes how a *flowing balance* (*Fliessgleichgewicht*) is possible, how the stability of structure can be assured even with the fluidity of change, how the complexity of the irregular shapes in the natural world around us can be comprehended. The new word is *fractals*, the "fantastic sequence of patterns within patterns—all similar without ever being identical." (Capra, p. 147) The shape of the whole is similar to itself at all levels of scale. Like a cauliflower. Or like snowflakes (Capra, p. 147). Or a reminder of the structure of an intimate autonomy? Each leans on or uses the other. Each remains autonomous while at the same time there is an intimate reciprocal use of each other.

Are my kitten and my pitbull naturally a sequence of patterns within patterns? *Transformation*, etymologically a derivative of the Latin *transformare*, does mean to change the shape or form of. Perhaps there is no intrinsic change but rather a reincarnation of a geometrical fractal hidden, a "stability of structure with the fluidity of change," split off or repressed until now. What a strange thought: my little sweet kitten and a pitbull! And is this what analysis is really all about? Is this what a process of becoming conscious entails, the unveiling of a fractal substructure? Is this *formation, transformation…*? Or, to use the Jungian term, *individuation*? Is this what the dream of the circumambulating lions becoming humans and reverting then back to lions ad infinitum touches on, too? But then they are not separate entities, each unto itself. Rather, there are layers within layers, forms within forms…fractals.

But this one of the four kittens was adapted and normal. Why her? Even if she can also remain the same, even if she can keep her own structure and also flow into yet another structural organization. I don't want her to change. I don't want her to assume a new shape, to reveal her pitbull structure shaping a quintessential part of her. She could then actually *be* a pitbull! Pitbulls are used and trained for illegal dog fighting in the United States. They've been known to attack and kill other animals as well as humans. We read such statistics as: "Attacks by pitbulls are associated with higher morbidity rates, higher hospital charges, and higher risk of death than are attacks by other breeds of dogs. … Strict regulation of pitbulls may substantially reduce the US mortality rates related to dog bites." (Bini, Cohn, Acosta, McFarland, Muir & Michalek, 2018)

Hypothetically, I've already stated that the kitten does not literally change. Perhaps a structure hitherto hidden or split off is unearthed. Perhaps she has always been a pitbull as well as a kitten; perhaps analysis is not primarily about transformation. Rather, analysis is a process of excavation, a disinterment to lay bare unrecognized and hidden fractal parts necessary to comprehend the complete in-dividual—as well as life itself. Perhaps our anaclitic regression has opened latent eyes in us or has reactivated the dragonfly eyes. Or the eyes of the blind kitten. Or the blind seer, Tiresias. We are then not viewing a new landscape, but instead we are uncovering; we are seeing more; we are becoming more conscious. With eyes that see a more differentiated landscape. With eyes that can unearth fractal entities, we can consciously choose between *kitten time* and *pitbull time*, between kitten energy and pitbull energy.[85] Indeed, we can actively encourage a dialectic communication, a third-space relating pattern. At times the pitbull and the kitten play with each other, they are normal and nice; at times they can use, they lean on each other; at other times, they bite and they scratch. Or both. Or all. And can I then consciously decide whether or not to enter the fray? And use Anna and my relating patterns as an outer mirror? The inner and the outer—and the outer and the inner—they are usually a two in one. And sometimes a one in two, of course.

The word

I've got to calm down before I continue to write about this. Using words as my own, my successful and my most common defense mechanism and means of centering this present scattered energy, words as my bridge to my newly discovered space of breath, words that now play with each other until they settle on a perceived fitting expression…and then they—and I—become rather cool, calm, and collected, perhaps even more common, more adapted. Or do the words use me?

The word, or perhaps any other creative tool, can tap a wellspring potentiating an eternal truth and activate the autopoietic process immanent in a system. I have mentioned the tree system: Its pattern is embedded in the acorn, branches, pine needles, and color of every tree. A *tree center* holds everything together while the pattern, the tree process, unfolds. Were I to extricate myself from some ego-control, were I able to midwife the word, it could perhaps birth itself inside its own system. That is, tap its own primordial chord, its prehistoric *primal word* (*das Urwort*). The poet says: "To be a poet, you have to hear the chords

---

[85] It is perhaps relevant to note that, more often than not, persons who commit egregious crimes are often the "normal, adapted" neighbors, about whom people confirm gentleness, normal, and adapted behavior; perhaps a bit introverted. But certainly not violent, one hears. To even conjecture that this sweet person could be an assassin, a murderer, is for most beyond belief!

of the primordial word and let it resound throughout the word you write down." (Hauptmann quoted in Campbell, 1959, p. 50)[86]

If, however, I relate to the word—and *use* the word—in a kind of ego-bound intellectual *gymnastic gyration*, if I do not also let the word *use* me, if the word and I do not play with each other, then I can fall into a narcissistic state of hypnotic revelry. The result is usually a mere fountain of seductively sparkly trivia.

Anyway, I do feel much better, much more anchored on earth, much more centered, much more real. Intellectual gymnastics, when the *word play* reaches viable conclusions, when I can *lean* on words that simply appear—a horizontal actualization from a vertical fractal—an *Urwort* connection? When these words dance and then settle into patterns of organization—a dialectic in itself—then my relationship with them weaves me into everything else, and I feel more contained, more secure. The inner and the outer, the upper and the lower…all are in intertwined patterns of relationship. All are fractals, the *language to speak of clouds*.

The pitbull and the kitten

Now I can return to the pitbull, to the kitten and her *unsplitting*, her becoming two in one, her *formation, transformation*. The kitten—and I—can assume that with this "rough beast," the "center can hold." For it is not only me as a partner in this dance but also the process itself that can settle ultimately into a delightfully attuned and constructively creative expression of relevant wisdom.

Conscious distance and autonomous closeness are key concepts to nurture. In the case of the relationship between the fourth kitten and the pitbull, the linguistically adept kitten could be an adequate referee. He could observe from a "scientific" distance both the play, the attuning of the opposition, between the kitten and the pitbull and note as well

---

[86] Hauptmann sagt: "Dichten heisst, hinter Worten das Urwort aufklingen zu lassen."

the words and their evolving pattern. They have to fit the system as the pine needles a pine tree or oak leaves an oak tree.

The challenge is also to ascertain whether or not the system, the reciprocal leaning, the weaving of the process of transformation, can hold. Perhaps because this fourth kitten is normal and adapted; perhaps she is not in need of transformation; perhaps she is therefore the one of the four to mirror her journey back to the other three and out to me and to the world. Perhaps normalcy and adaptability as patterns of organization are worthy of a respect I have never granted them, being enclosed myself in a quite protected, nonrelated, and implicitly naïve composition of narcissistic encasement. The kitten and the pitbull have known for a long time that they are both part of a network of relationships; they are parts woven together, rather than parts necessarily estranged and in opposition to one another. They are fractal parts of a dynamic web; they are contradictions of a higher/lower truth. And typically, they would play together, mutually lean on each other, they would dance together, and they would fight fiercely…together.

They themselves do not split off each other. The psyche splits the experience of the pitbull off because with a preverbal, early trauma, the infant's tiny ego is too endangered. There is no possible center to hold together anything traumatic or intense. Our conifer tree system with such a split would perhaps evolve without pine needles; perhaps instead with oak leaves. I evolve with a *false self*.

Molt 7: The egg [87]

The rupture previously described, together with the violent betrayal of Anna's health, cracks our egg-womb. I have come to terms with leaning

---

[87] Marie Louise von Franz, quoted in Edinger (1985, pp 184-185), claims: "Creation myths often begin with a cosmic egg…Father Heaven and Mother Earth….exist in a continuous embrace…in this state nothing can come into existence…there is no space for anything to grow between them….The first act of creation is therefore the separation of the divine couple…pushing them sufficiently apart so that a space is created for the rest of creation. This can be compared to the cutting apart of the egg."

on Anna and expecting her to be able to contain the tension of Parkinson's and me while being able to deal concomitantly with her own physical and mental energies. I have assumed that she can easily accommodate the pitbull. This idealized pattern is now shattered. This hope *hisses* presently, and I am more in touch with reality. And at the same time, I feel abandoned. Anxiety screams. I am alone again. The pitbull breaks out of the egg, he births himself.

My pitbull's face reflects suppressed, seething anger, which until now has been split off, hidden. Up until now I would not have been able to hold the pitbull's anger or his intense energy. Ironically perhaps, at the same time, I yearn for his seemingly innate ability to say "No," his ability to withstand intimidation, his indifference to the *polite pleasing* behavior pattern. All this I also admire. Perhaps I do not need to lean on Anna so much anymore. I can use the pitbull. My pitbull.

And I also have my fourth kitten, my normal adapted kitten. With her talent to come to terms with any given situation, the fourth kitten heralds the pitbull's entry. The system changes abruptly at this moment of bifurcation, and a new pattern suddenly appears as the pitbull energy becomes accessible. As a new participant in this circum-navigational voyage, as a significant part of the process, as a fractal of the normal kitten, or perhaps as a returned part of a pair of opposites previously split off from each other, the pitbull makes its appearance. I now can access the uncovered half of these oppositional forces; I can dance with his strength, his force, and I can perhaps contribute to the flow between him and the fourth kitten, while they together and apart—in their intimate autonomous relating pattern—can imbue me with this structural balance.

This is all quite interesting, and being able to play and to dance likewise with words has stabilized me. To be able to be still and wait, to be able to catch even a whiff of the word's own word (*das Urwort*) opens a door to feelings of awe, the Old Testament awe, an experience of wonder, accompanied by physical trembling and teardrops of fear (*Ehrfurcht, ehren-to honor und Furcht-fear*).

Chaos theory

At this time, it feels appropriate to return to the topic of chaos theory and to ask why certain aspects of this theory—with its words like *systems thinking*, or *autopoiesis*, or *bifurcation*, or *fractal*—is relevant to our voyage. Succinctly—and probably ridiculously too short to be a worthy explanation—there are two features of chaos theory that are significant for us. First, chaos theory picks up and elucidates a prime leitmotif of this voyage, namely, the concept of a unified duality or of an intimate autonomy. "All living systems are networks of smaller components, and the web of life as a whole is a multilayered structure of living systems nesting within other living systems—networks within networks." (Capra, 1996, p. 209) Secondly, systems thinking has made me realize that nature *does*. This is significant for me because I do not have to *ego-do* and fall into my old repetition pattern of desperate ego control, an old known pattern whose inevitable dualistic energy becomes narcissistic, desperately involved in succeeding rather than failing. Instead, I can then at least attempt to let myself be carried "on the wings of nature," on nature's *doing*.[88] Or my body's doing? Or on the ever-changing oceanic waters of the voyage?

My father, the architect, was not a systems thinker, nor did he ascribe to chaos theory when he emphasized that form generates the more important space. He did seem to recognize, however, that visual perception was the door to understanding organic form. And if my father—as well as the great English anthropologist Gregory Bateson—had read Goethe, they would have agreed with his conviction that "Each creature is but a patterned gradation [*Schattierung*]

---

[88] Relevant also for us is Goethe's contribution to the study of biological forms from a dynamic, development point of view. "He admired nature's 'moving order' [bewegliche Ordnung] and conceived of form as a pattern of relationships within an organized whole. Goethe writes, "Each creature is but a patterned gradation [Schattierung] of one great harmonious whole." Goethe breathed life into the word morphology, a word for me akin to transformation, but primarily in its dynamic quality. Morphology is not linear, nor is it circular, nor is it spherical. It is a system of relations; it is relational, structural. Etymologically, contextual comes from the Latin contextus—to weave together. (See Capra, 1996, pp. 4-35.)

of one great harmonious whole." (Bateson, 1972, p. 449) My father did recognize that form and space are a two in a one. Both of these fractal parts belong to one system. A "contradictory unity of both." (Giegerich, 1998, p. 130)

To return now to our kitten and the pitbull, they are both parts of one system. They are a two in a one. And if one of the two is cast off from ego consciousness, growth is arrested.

When the shell of the egg breaks, the pitbull slips into consciousness. Previously hidden spaces are accessible. Once-upon-a-time known energies are unleashed. These spaces once filled with disintegrating anxiety, with such threatening images that my mere trace of an ego feels existentially threatened, are in a process of transmutation. When this syntactical surge of consciousness breaks through, I gain further access to my very essence, my core, my hole-center, personal spirit or spark, my *chi* energy. The question remains, however, whether or not I can be this core energy. This question is tantamount to the inquiry: Can I be myself instead of continuing to identify with my defensive false self? My core energy was the original red that neither my mother nor the nurses could withstand.

In dreams I note corroborating reactions to this fledgling transformation. I feel an increasing certainty about the stability of the newly formed relating patterns, patterns reflective of the kitten and the pitbull's present togetherness. I recognize my own ego strength becoming more grounded, more anchored. These shifts all hint of a firmer core relationship. There seems to be a new center holding everything together.

Some dream contents show images of my facing danger, and instead of literally taking to the air and flying away, I refuse to be intimidated. Or the relative scarcity of earlier images of my house being invaded, or my being in danger of attacks. Violent criminals do not pursue me anymore. Certain dreams point to an increased reliance on my body. For example, in one dream I am on the top of a steep mountain and am being forced to ski down. But I have no skis. I am going to have to rely on myself and on my shoes. I start tentatively down the slope with feelings of doom that are quickly dispelled the moment both my legs and the shoes prove to be ample for the course. In another dream, an old wise woman gives green bricks to my son to build a new house. These dreams make my nights calmer; I sleep better, longer, more deeply. I have never before experienced such a paradigmatic shift. Both physically and psychically I note crucial reorganization and reshaping of patterns.

Anna's and my relating patterns

Anna arrives punctually this time. She appears normal and adapted—like my kitten. On the second day, however, she is suddenly overcome with such intense weakness, coughing, and lack of appetite that she goes to bed, where she remains for the following three days. My husband and I both consider taking her to the hospital. On the fourth day, she gets up and seems suddenly to be once again normal and adapted.

I, however, once more—but even more intensely than the last time—experience a violation of trust, a betrayal. Consciously, I feel shoved savagely and irreconcilably out of the nest and abandoned, while unconsciously I must have felt again the similar violent abuse as after my birth. Also, the leaning-on factor of our anaclitic therapy transmutes from my leaning on Anna to mutually shared moments. But alas, the strawberry-blonde infant in me is still too immature. She still needs to be able to lean on Anna—to use her. She still can not attach to the safety center inside, she still looks for Heinz Kohut's "love mirrored in the eyes of the mother" rather than viewing herself in herself or in me (Kohut, 1971). [89]

It is not a conscious decision on my part, but I must have felt such anger at Anna and desperation that I find myself withdrawing from any closeness. I remember films I have seen on attachment theories. The

---

[89] "Glanz im Auge der Mutter." Kohut defines these moments of positive mirroring in the mother's eyes as necessary for the infant's healthy development.

faces of infants are shown after being separated for the first time from the mother for two weeks, or whose mothers have looked at them "just for fun" with a "still face." You can view these infants in these films reacting with facial expressions of denial, desperation, and then slowly receding into another "space," "disappearing." The intensity of the pain is too much for a small ego to contain, and the psyche splits the suffering off. What is left is the false self that Winnicott describes. And an abiding terror of intimacy.

After a couple of days, Anna looks at me intensely and remarks: "Meredith, what is going on with you? I can't reach you anymore. You have closed yourself to me. Once again you seem to have become the Snow Queen."

With the words Snow Queen, I am instantly transported to our ranch in the Colorado mountains, where we always went for the three months in the summer to play, and in the winter to get our Christmas trees. With the words *Snow Queen*, images instantly throb through my blood and vault gleefully from cell to cell. Images I have known since our father had read Hans Christian Andersen's fairy tale "The Snow Queen" to us three children. Memories embedded in my body, a somatic experience yielding visions of the pine trees sparkling in their crystallized cloaks of hoar frost and this beautiful woman with long flowing hair covered with snowflakes, snowflakes of various sizes cascading around and off her body while she—like Ahab on ocean waters—sails on waves of whiteness from tree to tree. She sails from earth up to the sun in the heavens and then slides on the rays of the sun back down to her shimmering net of crystallized pine needles, back and forth and forth and back. Through every opening between the trees she dances and scatters fractals, flakes of snow like falling stars from a night sky, or drops of liquid crystal sliding down and up the rays of the sun. The Snow Queen! And, of course, true to my instant projected identification, seeing her is like looking into a mirror. I feel at home. My safety is affirmed, my protection confirmed, my repetition compulsion sustained. Once again from days long forgotten when my psyche split me off from my feelings to protect my very core. I am regressed back to my beginning—albeit this time consciously—reliving my birth. Once again, I am alone in a room. The door is shut. Once again, I am on the metal weighing scale, cold. I am slipping off.

It feels like the vertical split all over again. [90] I am home again!

The birth of the pitbull

But this time it is not the defensive split, (which will be elucidated and differentiated in Molt 2: The Split) but rather the offensive breaking of the egg: It is an autonomous, an aggressive I-Moment act, a bifurcation point. The pitbull breaks apart the shell and births himself. And I experience him attacking me physically. And I feel his anger as my own anger regarding Anna.

Perhaps he has been around for a couple of months now; perhaps in his new connecting relationship with me, he is enjoying a kind of revenge for having been ignored for so long. For months now, I have been experiencing a slicing pain in my right leg and in the left side of my neck. After X-rays and a consultation with my favorite medical doctor, the diagnosis is arthrosis. More physical limitation! That night I lie awake most of the night. As usual now, sudden insights lighten the bedroom with a soft but penetrating luminescence. I *know* that the pitbull has been attacking my body for years but now know that he can *come out* and that I can recognize and can accommodate his intensity and his aggressiveness. All I have been able to do up until now has been to defend against pitbull force by becoming the Snow Queen. Often, I

---

[90] This spiral-development, whereby one regresses again and again and each time advances in consciousness, mirrors the alchemical statement: Life consists of separatio and coagulatio, rhythmic, one and then the other. Only separated entities can unite, Jung points out. See C. W. Jung, Collected Works 12, paras 671 and 672. And this idea leads me to the Axiom of Maria, a precept in alchemy: "One becomes two, two becomes three, and out of the third comes the one as the fourth." It is attributed to third-century alchemist Maria Prophetissa, also called the Jewess, sister of Moses. Marie-Louise von Franz gives an alternative version thus: "Out of the One comes Two, out of Two comes Three, and from the Third comes the One as the Fourth." See Edinger, 1995, pp. 276-280.

freeze—or more aptly expressed, I become frozen, instead of the more usual fight/flight defense. I idealize her, I identify with her. I feel safe not feeling anything. The pitbull has been restrained in the shadows. Imprisoned without trial, he must make himself known somehow. His kind of shadow psychic energy manifests often autonomously. Clinically, the rage of the pitbull transmutes into psychosomatic attacks.

The Snow Queen thaws, and at this point it is all between the pitbull and me and the kitten and Anna, directly, unclouded; there are not so many defense mechanisms, not so many snowflakes keeping us apart, protecting me.

The pitbull has been/is my *Eros*, my life force. He offers me an access to red rage. The pitbull has become for me a validation of life's agency, of life's *life*. In contrast, however, the Snow Queen still remains present and persists in maintaining my addiction to *Thanatos*, to death, to my addiction to not change, to not feel, to be frozen, and at the same time, to desperately maintain my dualistic stance of always being right.

The Snow Queen, in her fractional crystallization of the archetypal image of the dismembering negative mother, drinks the red blood of the infant, eclipses its pulse of life. The blood assumes the pigment of silvery white. The infant—and then later the adult—feels no pain; she lives in splendid isolation on a beautiful, icy, crystal lake and reigns supreme in her absolute knowledge about what is right and what is wrong. Pure white is her color. White teems with all the colors and is empty at the same time. Like the whiteness of the whale, her whiteness is the "colorless all-color" because it is representative of the "great principle of light," the indicator of beauty as well as the frightening infinity of the universe (Schenk, 2001, p. 148).

The pitbull, on the other hand, quickens my spirit. I recall Mephisto's introduction to Faust explaining that his energy compels him to do evil, but he always ends up doing good. Illnesses like Parkinson's disease, or arthrosis, tend to deaden or mold into a statue. Recently, after fracturing six ribs and my sacrum, the pitbull has left me with osteoporosis, and with scoliosis, and for the first time, I experienced intense pain. While a pitbull is usually experienced as an evil attacker, instead, my body feels as if it has been catapulted into life and sparked with fire and Eros.

If I could trust nature more, if I would allow Eros—or the pitbull—more space in my life; if I could hear and believe the artist who paints trees and knows and recognizes the *good* in raw nature, the Snow Queen would have to bow to a greater force. The artist Emily Carr recognizes the inevitability—and the quality—of life's gifts. She writes:

Nothing can drown that force that splits rocks and pavements and spreads over the fields. ... No killing, no stamping down can destroy it. Life is in the soil. Touch it with air and light and it bursts forth like a struck match. Nothing is dead, not even a corpse. It moves into the elements when the spirit has left it, but even to the spirit's leavings there is life, boundless life, restless and marvelous, fresh and clean, God. (Shadbolt, 1987, p. 155)

Ironically, my kitten's fractal, the pitbull, births himself to keep me in life, to propel me into becoming real. Like Mephisto with Faust?

What causes this newly deepened dimension of instability? What tears the rupture open to an even more intense, more eruptive bifurcation? Why am I now given this shove into life?

Perhaps I have not been able to hold the center before now, and I could not allow the center to hold me. Perhaps I have been too terrorized to lean, to trust the other to hold me. I feel my anger at Anna subside; my anxiety recedes. Perhaps the journey with Anna, getting to know for the first time in my life what softness, what autonomous closeness and trust, are—these ever-so-intangible—yet felt and experienced—good-enough mother qualities; perhaps these all have transformed the shape, the structure of my vertical split into a horizontal split. Perhaps the anaclitic description of a preverbal wounding does not apply to me anymore! Perhaps somewhere, somehow in me—conceivably because I am older—there is now a "relentless desire to cross boundaries felt to be arbitrary constraints on the life of the human spirit." (Josey, 2013, p. 179) While at the same time, my tendency to let myself be deadened by Thanatos' forces, remains stubbornly assertive and persevering.

Now, when Snow Queen moments reign, for example in an exam, a frozen but consciously chiseled and seductively appropriate behavior takes over. The difference is—at the least most of the time—the Snow Queen is a conscious assistant. With Jung's "the only sin there is, is unconsciousness" ringing in my ears, the opposites of success or failure begin to play with each other. These two well-known dualistic forces become unglued, and their split energies shape-change into unified yet autonomous sparks of curiosity.

And so it was. And so it is. And so it will be?

Molt 6: Optimal oppositional friction

So, what do I do at this point? In my dream I have the delegated responsibility to tame the pitbull into not attacking me physically anymore, that is, psychosomatically. I have the responsibility not to project him out, whereby I can lose his strength, his vitality, and his self-confidence. Consequently, I am relegated to victim status—as often before in dreams. Also, I have the responsibility to not identify with him, to maintain my autonomy, as I've done with the Snow Queen. So how do I reach him?

I recall suddenly a possible meeting ground. At least a path that could lead me to a third-space encounter with him. I remember my body's reaction—a physical response— after attending to an inner active imagination a long time ago: I had just begun to teach at the Waldorf Schule in Frankfurt. Four conferences had been called to condescendingly criticize my manner of teaching. After school was over, I had been taken to a conference room, a large space where I was to sit in front of all of the schoolteachers and administration. They sat in a half circle, close to each other, a form from which I was excluded. After they had expressed various spurious accusations (like standing behind the students instead of always remaining in front), I suddenly saw them all dressed in black, and I felt like a witch on trial in Salem.

After the third conference when similar arrows were thrown at me, I went to my car and just sat there. My body was literally shaking. Suddenly, I remembered advice from my training analyst in Zurich: I should practice active imagination (a widespread Jungian technique) by speaking with a figure from one of my dreams.

At that time, I dismissed active imagination as kitsch, totally irrational, and ridiculous. I knew that Jung describes this method as the only way toward a direct encounter with the unconscious without the intermediary use of tests or dreams. At the end of his life, Jung remarked that passive imagination had been more or less understood by the world, unlike active imagination. In short, what was lacking was the active, ethical confrontation, the active entering of the whole person in the fantasy-drama (Hannah, 1981, pp. 1-13).

I sat in the car for a while and then I thought, why not try it? As I am in training at the Jung Institute and as I am there to learn to be a Jungian analyst, why not just see what it's like? Then I spoke with this dream figure, and five minutes later a gentle wind blew soothingly throughout my whole being. It was amazing. My body became quiet. I felt calm and centered. It was one of the experiences that converted me to analytical psychology, a psychological direction I had almost rejected as New Age, as kitsch, as a psychological route bound to crystals rather than to soul. My dream figure answered me!

With this memory and with the feeling of the softness of my body after the active imagination, I go to this third space of dialogue through the gates of this technique. The third space where the wind becomes gradually your own breath, a space that transports you often enough into a liminal place that harbors a dynamism of eternal time and infinite scope, a space where I stop *thinking*, where my ego lets go and waits for others to enter. I apperceive the pitbull; I let him in. He enters.

I am hit by current after current of air that seems to wash through me as a liquid breeze. I come to recognize that it isn't about the pitbull and me alone, but that any interchange with the pitbull implicates my sweet and normal, adapted kitten. These two are one. And they are also two. These two are intimately autonomous! The kitten is then also there.

Once again after a long absence from this entrance to a third space, I decide to ask Anna if she is willing to participate in an active imagination. I explain its importance: that it has to do with our relating pattern specifically and in general with an intimate autonomous pattern. I tell her that opposites—or twos like us—do emerge out of one *river*. The one river contains the two of the opposites. This is what Heraclitus meant by "No man ever steps into the same river twice." And the depth of this river is the depth of the soul. I recall his words "You cannot find the ends of the soul though you travelled every way, so deep is its logos." And together with Heraclitus' iconoclastic "War is both ruler and king...strife is justice...opposition brings concord," (Hillman, 1979, p. 25) the infinite value of frictional discord becomes clear.

The most important ingredient for friction is the two; the most essential ingredient for a relationship is the one. This sixth molt and the shedding of the repetition compulsion of forbidding rage-energy, of fearing red anger, marks a shift in consciousness. While wondering how the pitbull and I can ever adjust and attune our differences, I realize that we do not have to. We absorb them. Perhaps just by being near each other and engaging in dialogue or play or by engaging in conflict: by engaging in an optimal oppositional friction. Such a dynamic can be the strongest wind possible to breathe life into a relating pattern of calibrated intimacy and connecting autonomy.

Once again Indra's net spins its web of reality into my consciousness. I *see*—or the blind kitten sees—Indra weaving together the heavens and the earth, the humans and the animals, the conscious and the unconscious spaces, and then I watch...to be able now to see with the blind eye of the second kitten: the lens through which one is able to observe from the inside out rather than from the ego, the lens that renders the observer into an object as well as being the subject, the lens that opens the space to apperception. The third space becomes once again an experience along with its being a notional conception. I recall once again Winnicott's discovery of a path out of the welded *inner and outer* into

[a] third area of human living, one neither inside the individual nor outside in the world of shared reality... [an] intermediate area of experience [that] starts with children playing. ... When [their] toys recede into the background, there remains the residue of the inventiveness that generates art and the curiosity that drives science. (Davis & Wallbridge, 1981, pp. 45-66; Jones, 2002, p. 45)[91]

With the consciousness of an artist, a scientist, or any creative person, there can be an inclination to gather the parts together and then *let them go*: let them play, dance, experience their unity and their difference, know their optimal oppositional friction, find the dialectical movement between the opposites. Instead of the experience of split opposites, the experience of the process and force of systems thinking becomes more pertinent. A playful dialectic in the third space can reveal a more relevant reality. I suggest to Anna that we can open up to the emptiness of nothingness, to a speaking which evokes rather than spells out or nails down...a speaking that reveals the unspeakable, yet reveals it in such a way that by the very revealing, it preserves its secret. ... Why is the moment of secret and silence necessary at all? ... because the soul IS the contradiction and difference (here between speaking and silence, revealing and concealing)...it is the dialectical logical life playing between the soul's opposites. (Giegerich, 1998, pp. 32-38)

Anna wants to take part in this experiment of active imagination. Having taken part in such a deep process as our anaclitic therapy, inevitably she also has been affected. She remarks that she is curious.

With a lighted candle on the floor in the middle of my practice, with the sun shining through my windows, its light breaking the prism of various stones and showering the room with colors and—like the egg—opening to a many-hued reality, I invoke the following actors...

---

[91] For Winnicott, the creation of culture begins with children playing.

and then we wait...receptive, we wait for words, for silences and secrets, and for action...and we are intrigued and a bit fearful.

Myself, Anna, the fourth kitten, the pitbull, the blind kitten, the physically delicate kitten, the linguistically talented, archaeologist kitten as scribe, and the Snow Queen. *Ach!* And Parkinson's disease.

September 16, 2013

Active Imagination

Cast:
WK - Weak Kitten
M - Meredith
PD - Parkinson's Disease
P - Pitbull, Butch
A - Anna
Kit - Normal, adapted fourth kitten
BK – Blind Kitten
SQ - Snow Queen

Summary: The weak, delicate kitten serves gingerbread and tea. Meredith speaks to the pitbull and expresses her need for his strength and his self-assertive aggression. At first, he refuses to talk with her. He states that he has often feared that his anger would take possession of him and does not want to contaminate her. They have all to meet in the third space and play. The pitbull talks for a long time with the kitten part of him, with our normal, adapted kitten, the fourth one. She takes on some of his fire; he shares with her his yearning to belong, to feel normal. Meredith exclaims with joy that she can already feel some of the characteristic qualities of the pitbull and of the adapted kitten and of the calmness of Anna. The blind kitten remains silent throughout. When asked, she replies that she "does not feel a thing, that she has nothing to say," that she is waiting. Toward the end of this active imagination, Anna gives the pitbull the responsibility of becoming more accessible to us all and of protecting us when needed. He is so moved, he feels so perceived; an important part of his essence is finally recognized. He gets tears in his eyes. The Snow Queen *dissolved herself in her own water*, she is there and not-there; she is now an energy *in potentia*. When needed she is willing to be available. And as for Parkinson's Disease:

PD: I am not even invited to attend this conversation! What do they think I am? An empty nothingness? Or, on the other hand, perhaps they are dealing exclusively with the unconscious. And I am certainly a conscious aspect of Meredith's life! This conceptually filigreed differentiation between the conscious and the waters of the unconscious is, of course, relevant. Even now I am intrigued by the pitbull and his "evil" energy.

I think I'll just hang around and observe. If neither Meredith nor Anna notices me, I'll grab Meredith and *catch* her in my usual cruel fashion. It's called "tough love."

Actually, when I think about it, I miss her. I wonder if she misses me?

WK: I have brought the gingerbread, plates, and forks. Anyone can take what she wants.

When—and if—she or he wants something.

M: At this moment, I do not feel any anxiety regarding you, pitbull. I would like to sense in myself at least a little bit of your steadfastness and your firm strength. If I could touch this in me, perhaps I would not cry so easily. I do not like to be overwhelmed and have to cry when I do not want to. My mother always said: "Meredith, do not be so emotional." Anna says to me: "You were born close to water." (*Du bist nah am Wasser gebaut.*) My crying is me and not-me. I feel sort of funny…

P: (Silently. To himself.) Meredith, I do not feel like *giving* you anything. As a matter of fact…is it a fact? Anyway, what I mean is that I cannot *give* you something. Perhaps I could open myself more and then with a dialectical communication, an *optimal friction* could set in. You might feel this friction and thereby interiorize it. I could then begin to become a more conscious part of your energy.

But actually, when I look at you suffering because of me, and when I perceive what you are going through, then it makes me feel sad. But it also makes me aware of a potential source of dialogue. We are so different. You are a *victim* of mine, you feel impotent. I feel strong and in control of me and of my life—perhaps I am too confident, too sure of myself. But exactly these *opposites* can open a door to dialogue. Our radical differences are like the two sides of the same coin…I've heard you humans say: "Let's play and see what happens." I wonder how you—and I—and the others—will get along?

P: (looking at Anna) What I'd like to have from you, Anna, is your ability to *feel*, or to *know*, how somebody else is feeling. I am always so full of red anger that this feeling—and this dominating color—runs away with me and I lose the relationship with others.

A: I suggest that you stay close to me. I am going to feed you, pet you, play with you, and you can lay your head in my lap, and when your anger comes, then let me know, and I will touch you, and we will see what happens.

Kit: Dear Anna, I know what normal and adapted is, and it is definitely not normal and adapted for a pitbull to put his head in your lap and for you to pet him. Even though he is a part of me, actually, I do not like him. I could imagine that he could bite you when you least expect it. In my opinion, you are too naïve and too optimistic.

A: It might sound naïve, but I anticipate his attacks and have already planned how to protect myself with leather wristbands, for example. I do know how risky, how dangerous it is to allow the pitbull to get this close to me. It is, however, the only possibility of altering our relating pattern. The unpredictability of his behavior I am fully conscious of. But I don't have any other alternative. I want things to be different between us.

M: But Anna, you do not have to go to all that trouble if you would just be realistic and see him for what he is: a pitbull. Just look at his face, you can see anger and disdain. We have to take him for what he is. Actually, we have to approach him very slowly and then see how he reacts.

A: If you look through the anger and the disdain, you will realize how much he has suffered. That is why he is so angry. He has been ignored and despised and has always been pushed away. It is important to realize that his firmness is an innate part of him and can contain intensity if he is conscious enough and can anticipate his inclination to explosive affect. And besides, if his anger does run away with him, that is also still OK. We can anticipate it and be prepared for it. I can talk with him, I can touch him. We can…

P: I am sorry to interrupt, I do not mean to be impolite, but you are all daft. You are ignoring me as if I were not here. You are speaking about me instead of to me. I would like to tell you something about myself, which is—as we have already noted—also something about both of you. We all emerge out of the same source.

1) To you, dear Kit, I have my firmness and steadfastness from you, because you are normal and adapted. But you are also boring. You need some fire, some intense energy, perhaps even some Eros from me! Perhaps conscious optimal friction would ignite you so you could flow more.

2) Meredith, as I've already pointed out, I cannot give you any of my steadfastness or firmness. No one can do this. But if you are willing to stay close to me, then you will automatically get it through osmosis. That is what our relating pattern, our intimate autonomy, is all about. Inevitably you take on colors of the person you are in relationship with. I assume what you want is to be able to go into yourself in order to find a place of peace instead of the terrifying hole which you still too often fall in to. You were not born with this hole. Try to go back to a time before your birth. That was the space where we were all together, we were one with nature, with the earth and with the heavens, and at the same time we were all different from one another. There was no hole. There was a structure, a pattern, and the network: a natural individuality and a natural togetherness, a *two in a one,* so to speak. Actually, that is

the way it always has been and ever shall be. Recognition is the key word. Consciousness!

3) Anna, unfortunately, I have to admit that you are right. It is realistic that on one hand

4) you offer me love and understanding, but also you are wise enough to protect yourself in case I endanger you. It is obvious that you have understood at least parts of the reality of good and evil. Isn't it boring for you to always be right?

A: To always be right would mean that I am, that my ego is always right, that I never make mistakes, that I am never wrong. No, what I mean is seeing everything through the lens of a third space. This means for me that somebody puts something in the middle of this third space, in this labyrinth of mirrors, like a word or a sentence for example. Or this someone puts herself into the space. And then all we do is watch and see what happens. Something will happen. The other person will or will not take this word out, and something new will arise—and that is not boring. Words are wellsprings. Words ignite. As does the silence of a well, of emptiness…Or when someone is willing to make herself vulnerable by exposing her *true* self. And waits to see what happens. This process obviates dualism.

M: Let's stop for now. I want to try to *eat* all we've talked about. I want to try to recollect certain points:

1) I do not feel any object constancy. That means that you all probably will not stay with me and I will then fall into my hole.[92]

---

[92] Object constancy. Third year and beyond. An internalization of the image of the mother. At this point, a child no longer really needs the mother's presence. He can hold the image of her inside while she's away. She can use an object like a toy to supply comfort in her absence. If we were to use our language, we would say that the child was now able to be autonomous, i.e., she can feel alone, when she is with another person; and she can feel intimately attached, when she is alone. According to Winnicott, this is an achievement that forms "a basis for life…because the state of being alone is something which (though paradoxically) always implies that someone is there" (Winnicott, quoted in Davis & Wallbridge, p. 40).

2) As for you, Butch, that is your name isn't it? Perhaps all the time you have been making fun of us, and when we turn our backs to you, you will attack and laugh.

3) Ach, what I really feel like doing now is to leave all this serious stuff and to concentrate only on the moving light of the candle and the delicious gingerbread.

4) And you, dear blind kitten, O'wise one, you have not said anything. I would like to know what you are thinking about all of this.

BK: (We waited but there was merely a loud silence.)

A: I do feel the need to say that I do see you, Butch, differently than Meredith. I trust and I believe that when you want to, you are able to assume the responsibility that we would like to give to you. You have yearned for such a long time to be in a space where you feel perceived, where you feel like you belong, where you can be in relationship, and where you can be a responsible person. You are now in such a space. As a matter of fact, you remind me of the sweet adapted kitten!

P: (With tears in his eyes): That is exactly what I had to hear, that you find me worthy of being able to be responsible. You assume I can do it. Your words tame my pain of having been an outsider for so long. You offer an opportunity to step into the silence often surrounding my appearance and provide a dash of friction—as well as protection as needed. Thank you, Anna.

Intermission

PD: I've waited. I've been patient. But now I've had enough! Regretfully, I was not invited to this get-together. Even though I am already here.

All of you seem to be trying to forget me, to repress me, to obliterate me into a nothingness. After all this talk about an intimate autonomy, not one of you is willing to make themselves vulnerable enough to get into this relating pattern with me. And a robust vulnerability is the key to autonomy! I cannot believe, that after all our work that none of you seem to know this.

I want to invite each and every one of you to consciously wake up to this fact that if you let me in, you are vulnerable to my attacks. But if you don't let me in, if you repress my *evil* existence, then all the attempts to relate to anything intimately and autonomously at the same time have failed. And it then becomes probable that I am going to have to graciously but violently interrupt this nice, cute little scene once again.

And Meredith, especially you! You have been able not merely to feel at the mercy of my whims. I thought you have attained a maturity whereby you can accept this vulnerability and even enjoy the autonomy won from being so *naked*. Especially from you, I feel so disappointed, so angry, so hurt, and so forgotten.

M: I really don't know where to begin. I do apologize. Obviously, I just take you for granted now. And I forget to relate to you as if you were *real*. I've become so accustomed to your *face*, to your attacks, to your newly experienced gentleness and willingness to relate to me in our aforementioned pattern, that I...I...just forgot you! I began to just take you for granted. It's unbelievable that such a thing can happen! It is like childbirth: It hurts so much, but then we forget the pain and have more children. But we have the child, whom we don't forget. And you—or perhaps more specifically, our relating pattern is the child. And I do feel so sad...and superficial... and scared... It reminds me of the 13th fairy in "The Sleeping Beauty." She was not invited to the christening of the new baby and placed a revengeful curse on the princess and the family.

PD: I do not want revenge. Nor will I forgive. To just forget me, to merely blank out my existence is perhaps almost tantamount to disregarding *evil*. To ignore evil is self-destructive! Quite a dangerous and even an immoral tendency. For the world, as well as for each individual. But I will strive for reconciliation between us. I am willing to try once again. I do like you, you know. But please, do try to not shut out the evils of life. They—like I am—are facts. We are not wraiths emerging out of mists arising from the *hisses* of hope. We are facts of life…and of death. Remember!

Molt 5: The dragonfly nymph
(Mitchell & Lasswell, 2005, pp. 56, 57, 67, 69)[93]

I am pregnant. I, the *child* in the anaclitic relationship with Anna as the *good-enough mother,* am pregnant with her, with the *mother,* and with myself. That sounds quite bizarre, doesn't it? Perhaps even stranger still, is that I feel pregnant with the energies of all the participants in the recent active imagination. It is a weird, a foreign feeling, to experience faint flutters of dragonfly wings together with the muted yet firm growls of the pitbull. The sudden appearance of the pitbull (to be confirmed by Meredith) as a partner in a relating pattern still vibrates throughout my body. And to surmise that "they" are determining structural changes instead of commands being issued by my brain to my body. It is a physical force—or a psychic force—wresting power from my brain, yet it feels more abstract than any other experience, for example, of being caught by Parkinson's. Something has happened. Something quite unfamiliar. Did the words of our active imagination conjure up this "pregnancy"?

For the quality of presence of the pitbull I am the most grateful. His strength, his force, and his fire are noted. Does the friction generated due to the oppositional energy of the sweet kitten plus

---

[93] "Our knowledge of dragonfly taxonomy begins with understanding both dragonfly development and morphology (form and structure). Dragonflies have two very separate phases of their lives: the larva (also known as nymph) or immature phase and the adult. The transformation from immature insect to adult can be gradual…or it can be extreme. … Metamorphosis may proceed over a fairly long period of time, such as over a winter. … Although eons old, the transformation of the aquatic larva to the aerial adult is still a marvel of biology. … Like the birth of a child, once the process starts, it becomes inevitable."
Is this experience a mirror of my 'work' with Anna?
See also my article "Illness as an Illusion of Misfortune" (2009).

Anna's concentrated calmness make this possible? I feel vibrations of the playful autonomies of them all. Echoes of their joyful enthusiasm along with their gasps of pain and silent screams…all of these I can feel and hear. Now I do not merely *perceive* them; I *know them*.[94]

Digesting the active imagination

A few days before Anna leaves again for Germany to return in six weeks, I am deeply embedded in my usual early ritual of trying to extract myself from my bed. According to all neurological research, Parkinson's disease results when there is a lack of communication from the brain to the body. The body remains paralyzed until this transmission is launched with the help of dopamine plus physical movement. Initially, every morning, I remain on my left side, unable to get up. I can, however, usually move my right arm up and down, and shift my feet back and forth. And I can breathe deeply and I can consciously withdraw ego-doing. I try to accord an equal amount of time and energy to the active *doing* and the receptive *being*. It is most difficult for me to relax and let my body *be* from the inside instead of concentrating on my arm's *doing* from the outside. Images of the gingerbread being flipped upside-down and downside-up dart about in my mind when I succeed in *being*. And from this space there is usually the spark—a Billy Elliot spark—that initiates the parting between me and the bed. But this spark comes from a relaxed position, from extricating myself from ego-control, from allowing myself to be the gingerbread and be turned upside-down.

Gradually, after taking dopamine and doing gentle gymnastics for about 1½ to 2 hours, I can feel a slight quickening of energy in the upper middle of my stomach area, the region where I feel my *chi* is located. If I can *touch* the vibration and contact the screaming silence there, then my whole body can begin to move, and I hear sounds like

---

[94] Once again, from the Apocrypha of John, the Apostle writes Christ's teachings, I recall the words that Christ teaches: If I am a lamp for you, you can perceive me. If I am a mirror for you, you can know me.

the fortissimo part of a symphony. I am on my way out! It is exhilarating. And often I think: This contact between the upper and lower body parts is more important than the drug-induced communication between my brain and my body. This moment of physical awakening is like being kissed by Aphrodite, perhaps akin to what Galatea feels when she suddenly melts into life.

This morning is different. I wake up as usual, but along with the "symphony," there is an image, an image other than that of the upside-down gingerbread, an image that darts around in the same space of the *chi* energy, an image mirroring the fossilized dragonfly larva that my husband gave me some years ago for a birthday present. Unlike the actual dragonfly larva, however, my larva/nymph is enclosed in a silvery white uteruslike spherical globe. Is this an introjection of a transformed Anna? Is she gestating in this womblike globe in me? Are all the members of this voyage, the dream figures as well the figures of our active imagination, likewise in this globe? What could this mean for me? And for Anna? And for us? Is the image of the white nymph the baton, the downstroke, to begin the symphony? Does the image of the white dragonfly nymph constellate a third space where an optimal oppositional friction dances in my brain, my body, and all the players in the active imagination into a third space? It feels like the direction of communication is now almost 90 percent my body to my brain, or my interiorized brain and my body and my ego together. What are the parts and the wholes? Indeed, can the spark to life originate in my body? Transmission is then the opposite of the previous trajectory. Or is this experience part of the combined optimal oppositional friction at which point the question or the origin of the communication becomes irrelevant? The *is* of the experience just is.

This does raise additional questions, and they deserve attention. But first I feel compelled to at least attempt to communicate what I have been experiencing since Anna's last departure.

Anna's and my separation

I sit in the car and see Anna step into the airport's revolving door; I watch the door suck her into the building. There is a loud crack, a crack like the opening of an egg. For the first time, a sadness, a deep feeling of mourning seizes me. Simultaneously, I want to leap into the air like Billy Elliot at the end of that impacting movie. Billy is 11 years old when he auditions at the ballet school. When he is asked what he feels while dancing, he replied: "I disappear. ... I become electricity." Years later as the Black Swan in Pyotr Ilyich Tchaikovsky's ballet, *Swan Lake*, we see him entering the stage and suddenly—with perfect form, molding his body into living beauty—he becomes a spark of physical eternity, embodied joy, crystallized bliss, and then his body seems to take over and, in a carefully finely tuned flash of music, like a shooting star, he whirls up into the heavens. We do not see his reappearance onto the stage floor but this return to earth and subsequent similar leaps are assumed.

This freedom, this sensual *disappearing* and at the same time knowing that I will *appear* again, I have never known before. Giving a lecture or simply being seen, I become filled with such anxiety that I desperately hold on, while experiencing a kind of split. Part of me seems to just take off on its own. My voice continues to speak, but *I* am somewhere else. From some other place I listen to my own voice. If Billy Elliot had had such a split, he couldn't have disappeared, he couldn't have "become electricity." His whole being makes this leap, not just part of him. His whole being becomes electricity, not just a part of him. Leaving Anna at the airport and feeling the wetness of the tears rolling down my cheeks, I experience at the same time a joy never touched before. A quiet, still joy. A deep, Beethoven's Ninth Symphony, "Ode to Joy" (*An die Freude*) kind of joy. Not the yippee, yippee variety. I know that the hole in me has been at least partially filled. I know that I—like Billy—am sort of whole for the first time in my life! I've never felt so firm or so held. Until now I've never grasped, I've never been able to sense, Faust's need to know what holds the world together from the inside. In Goethe's *Faust,* in his famous first major speech, Faust exclaims that he is sick and tired of dealing with *words, with philosophy, law and medicine and unfortunately also theology.* He wants to be able to recognize—to sense—what inner forces are holding the world together.[95]

I am held together by this nymph, by this white nymph, by something that does not "hold together" while it holds together. The hole has been filled with this energy, a structural pattern, which is Anna's and my relationship, attended by the friction of the optimal oppositional relating of all *of us.* I feel like a dynamic flow of perpetual movement. Anna flies away and leaves herself in me. Anna and I are together and not together. We have dissolved into living paradoxes, into…it feels like a space of nothing and everything. An intimate autonomy! A two in a one.

…I could imagine that this sounds quite absurd. I sense a need, therefore, to tend to more earthly matters for a while, not to leave Billy Elliot hovering in the heavens as a detached form of crystallized beauty, but rather to assume that he lands on earth again and is busy with matters such as what he should eat before the next performance.[96] And I want to look at a landscape of trees, of leaves and grass, instead of lingering in suspension between clouds and misty mountains far away. I want to *earth* any concept that I have left hovering in hazy abstractness; I want to be able to facilitate a relationship between the most beautiful and the most profane.

What does it mean to be "pregnant with Anna"? How does she "get inside" of me? Or the question regarding the split? Vertical or horizontal? Or what is anaclitic therapy anyway? Even though I have

---

[95] Ich habe nun, ach! Philosophie,/ Juristerei und Medizin,/ Durchaus studiert, mit heissem Bemuehn./ Da steh'ich nun, ich armer Tor,/Und bin so klug alswie zuvor! …Dass ich erkenne, was die Welt/Im Innersten zusammenhaelt,/ Schau' alle Wirkenskraft und Samen,/ Und tu' nicht mehr in Worten kramen. (Faust, lines 355-359; 382-385, my translation.)

[96] I would recommend this film, both for the scene I described as well as for the portrayal of the plight of coal miners in England as a contemporary political statement. Billy Elliot is a 2000 British drama film written by Lee Hall and directed by Stephen Daldry. Set in north-eastern England during the 1984-85 coal miners' strike, it stars Jamie Bell as 11-year-old Billy, an aspiring dancer dealing with the negative stereotype of the male ballet dancer; Gary Lewis as his coal miner father; Jamie Draven as Billy's older brother; and Julie Walters as his ballet teacher.

touched on anaclitic therapy, I feel able now to pass on experiential information about the therapy's healing potential. Experience is so much more *golden and green* than theory! And the color white? What is so singular about this color? Perhaps the whiteness of the nymph subsumes the nucleus, the summary of the voyage:

> In a new Third Space where the volatile combines with the fixed…where the Two become One. But not by joining, not by living them as oscillating alternatives, not by compensating one with the other. They have become One because they have lost their literal pulls. And they have lost their oppositional tension, because our attention is on their relations (rather than on their substantiality), the movement between them…. (Hillman, 2009, pp. 40, 41, 43)

As discussed in chapter 42 of Melville's *Moby Dick*, "The Whiteness of the Whale," it is the incantation of the color white which quickens (Melville, 1847/1967, pp. 161-170). White refracted reveals a multitude of hidden colors. A many in a one.

Molt 4: The pregnancy

> "The transformation of the aquatic larva to the aerial adult Is still a marvel of biology. … Like the birth of a child, once the process starts, it becomes inevitable" (Mitchell & Lasswell, 2005, pp. 67, 69).

And like any system, the process is autopoietic. Like the acorn once planted unfolds according to its system. My "pregnancy," a living structural process now implanted inside me, unfolds according to its endemic intimate autonomy pattern, its two-in-one network. Unlike our acorn, however, the autonomy inside me is an intimately unified multiplicity of Anna and of me and the others—and of a dragonfly. And of the kitten and the pitbull?

Part Three

The placenta

The placenta is the third-space connector to the uterine wall, to my white spherical globe, to my body. Through the quickening spark of the *third-space placenta*, the process unfolds. This procedure sustains the living quality of the nymph, the *unified duality* (*geeinte Zweiheit*) of Anna and me, as well as of the additional members of our conversation. Various functions of the placenta include nutrient uptake, waste elimination, and gas exchange via my blood supply; it is the conduit for oxygen and nutrients, and for special hormones important during pregnancy. The placenta also provides a reservoir of blood for the nymph, to be used, for example, in the case of hypotension.

The word *placenta* comes from the Latin word for "cake," due to its flat shape. Even though the placenta is actually formed from the two components of the fetus/larva or nymph and that of the mother, it assumes the combined functions mentioned, a unified duality serving life. In pre-Roman languages of tribal cultures, the placenta is often referred to as the "little mother," or "grandmother." In German, placenta is a "mother-cake" (*Mutterkuchen*).

My nymph—this being that is me and not-me—is now being held by the globe, the uterinelike vessel, and is nourished by the organ connecting the nymph to its perimeter, by the placenta, the inter-regional third space. The third-space placenta inhabits a kinship or affinity to Jung's bilateral point: I recall this place where the opposites play and dance until they become a "vessel in which what was one thing and now another floats vibrating, so that the painful suspension between opposites gradually changes into the bilateral activity of the point in the center." (Jung, 1971, para. 296) In my case, the "opposites" feel as if they are the upper and the lower body parts. In between is the latent *chi* waiting to be sparked into life.

The placenta vibrates with the timelessness of eternity while dancing a fugue with the present; the placenta is as spaceless as infinity while offering the containment of firm, tenacious holding. The placenta hums with a joyful equanimity while harboring death's last breath and life's first gasp.[97] A place of steadily sustained movement interrupted intermittently by the friction of an optimal oppositional engagement.

The aquatic larva's transformation to the aerial adult dragonfly depends to a large degree on the placenta's pulsing blood and life-granting oxygen transmogrifying structurally from the placenta to the wings. I recall my astonishment at my knowledge of the physical, the mitochondrial life-giving veins of the dragonfly's wings not being discordant with my experience of the wings' whispered beauty.

The wings of the dragonfly appear to be translucent sheets of shimmering mica. Seen through the lens of an artist, the mitochrondrial veins chisel geometrical patterns and transform the wings into ancient tiny mirrors recalling images of mirror rooms in the Taj Mahal – or perhaps, upon reflection, golden metallic squares and circles of a Klimt painting comes to mind.

The beauty and apparent fragility of the dragonfly often belie the physical strength and versatility. Along with their artistic etching, the veins channel the oxygen and blood that lend the dragonfly her unique physical adeptness to hover, and then suddenly to dart at a speed that can tease the perception of a dragonfly into a possible illusion. (Oenning-Hodgson, 2009, pp. 50-51)

Perhaps the wings of the dragonfly are reflected in the placenta. Perhaps the wings of the dragonfly dissolve themselves into the placenta. Or the wings of an angel, its beauty, and its terror. I return once again to Rilke:

Denn das Schöne ist nichts
als des Schrecklichen Anfang, den wir noch gerade ertragen,
und wir bewundern es so, weil es gelassen verschmäeht,
uns zu zerstören. Ein jeder Engel ist schrecklich.
(Rilke, 1992)[98]

---

[97] In Faust I, in the Prologue in Heaven, the angel Gabriel's description of Earth aptly describes this placenta space. There one experiences both the ecstasy of the light of paradise and the terrorizing empty depth of the darkness of night. (Es wechselt Paradieseshelle mit tiefer schauervoller Nacht, 253, 254.)

[98] : [Author's translation]"...for Beauty is nothing more than the beginning of a terror/which

When the form, the shape, the skin of the placenta begins vibrating with coagulating blood, with dancing cells, when the *chi* energy becomes vital with life's spark, my symphony begins. Subsequently, with the dragonfly darting hither and thither, we have left the world of the fetus and have thrown off the confinement of the uterus, we have digested autonomously the gifts of the placenta; we have emerged. And "once this process starts, it becomes inevitable." And the initial holding-task of the *inside placenta* is given over to the *outside mother*. Once again, opposites, like the upside and down parts of the gingerbread, are busy trying to find the other's music—and more. They have perceived their functions to be the cutting edges of a common interface, where the *upside* and the *down* are stretched into a third space of autonomous yet intimate chemically abrasive juices flowing in and out of each other. First, a cacophony of musical notes, of twos, of threes, of fours, and then the attainment of the crescendo of a paradoxical many-in-one. A space alive. A *hiss* space. A once-upon-a-time virginal space now opened for gestation. A dynamic space of relating.

The good-enough mother scaffolding

For D. W. Winnicott, observed facts are a reality, and "theories were the human stammer towards grasping the facts" (Winnicott, 1971, pp. 9-10). While Melanie Klein's description of a preverbal infant may include the babe dwelling in a *paranoid/schizophrenic* space, or Freud's focus on the repetition compulsion in terms of a death instinct could describe moments of a preverbal or pre-ego infant's anxiety, such theories are interesting but fade in comparison to "life's golden tree":

> *"All theory, dear friend, is gray.*
> *But life's golden tree is green."*
> (Goethe, 1806/1992, lines 2038-2039)[99]

---

for the first time we are able to contain,/And we hold it in awe because it calmly and full of contempt refuses to destroy us. Every angel is terrifying." The relevant portion of Rilke's "The First Elegy" is located in Appendix A-11.

[99] Grau, teuerer Freund, ist aller Theorie,/ Und gruen ist des Lebens goldner Baum.

THE HISS OF HOPE

Winnicott writes at the end of his life, after working with Melanie Klein, Anne Freud, and Susan Isaacs, and after going through psychoanalytical training, that "direct clinical observations of babies…have indeed been the main basis for everything that I have built into theory." (Winnicott, 1971, p. 19) For the preverbal newborn, he recognizes *holding* to be the sine qua non, to succor the "native honesty which so curiously starts in full bloom in the infant, and then unripens to a bud," if the infant has not been held by a good-enough mother. The poet describes it:

The baby new to earth and sky,
…But as he grows he gathers much
And learns the use of 'I' and 'me',
And finds 'I am not what I see,
And other than the things I touch.'
So rounds he to a separate mind
From whence pure memory may begin
As through the frame that binds him in
His isolation grows defined.
(Tennyson, 1850)[100]

Through Anna's holding, I become defined. Through our relating, through Anna's baby whispering, through our determination and commitment to be part of this, our voyage, our odyssey both in and out of water, through our ability to both be in a third space replete with infectious good humor and empathy and simultaneously to observe and to differentiate between physical and psychic symptoms, between hysterical features and phenomenological experiences, between projection and observation, yet primarily perhaps through our loving perseverance and dedication to our intersubjective task, we have together begotten this intrapsychic white nymph and the enclosing globe with its bilateral placenta.

I just reread what I wrote in this molt and, true to my design of an intimate autonomous relating pattern between the mists of distant

---

[100] The full text of "In Memorium: 45" is located in Appendix A-5.

mountains and the defined outlines of accessible oak trees, I will once again highlight and unravel three potentially nebulous words or concepts.

The words *introjection, real,* and *pregnant* remain perhaps ambiguous.

Introjection

How does an introjection happen? Is introjection concomitant to eating a piece of the upside-down gingerbread and digesting it? How do Anna, of Anna and me, and the dragonfly become interiorized?

It is a common feature of most close relationships that we catch ourselves unconsciously picking up words of the other, beginning to move like the other in little ways, wearing scarves when we never had considered it before. Or, I remember learning how to ski by skiing behind my talented nephew. In this case, the latest neurological research identifies *mirror neurons*, responsible for human empathy and imitation, to have perhaps caught the rays of the snowy mountain sun and then fired my ability to go speeding down steep inclines, even black paths, remaining close to the back tips of his skis. By myself, I never would have even attempted such a challenge.[101]

An additional example of unconscious introjection is the moment when the white nymph as the dragonfly larva and I become one while also remaining two. The image of the white globe containing the nymph—like any image—seems to drop into my line of vision, like from a twilight space akin to a dream space. For me, it is a moment of consciously opening a door of receptivity and catching the image catapulting in. Often there are too many instead of too few. It is a typological character trait of mine that I cherish and understand these abounding creations most often as objective entities, as realities present in the liminal interface between worlds. There is a necessary

---

[101] See Huffman, Younger & Vanston, 2010, p. 169.

unfathomability in this receptivity zone, which I likewise cultivate and honor as real. For Jung, these are likewise *living moments*. Once again, I recall his words:

> We all have an understandable desire for crystal clarity, but we forget that in psychic matters we are dealing with processes of experience...a re-experiencing...of that twilight which we can learn to understand only through inoffensive empathy, but which too much clarity dispels. (Jung, 1982, Bd. 13, para. 199)

This image of the white nymph is a gathering together of introjected fugitive fuguelike pieces both from my voyage with Anna as well as the generous and loving accompaniment reality of my husband and of the dragonfly, which has been my constant spirit animal/insect since 2008.

Real

Introjection occurs for the most part unconsciously or neurologically. The pregnancy is real and is at the same time an illusion, in the sense of Winnicott's statement that the reality principle is "the arch-enemy of spontaneity, creativity, and the sense of Real" (Winnicott, 1971, p. 57). But illusion or not, the white globe, the nymph, and the others are in me and seem to have also claimed the energy of the *chi*. For when I am going through my ritual of freeing myself from my bed, I have noticed that if I consciously send my breath to the globe long enough and rhythmically enough, the globe begins to send soft silvery bell sounds out, whose vibratory dynamic seems to awaken the *chi* and my upper and lower body come together faster. That is real.

Pregnancy

This pregnancy has occurred due to the interactions between Anna and me, as well as the active imagination dialogues with other voyage members. I am pregnant—or I am filled with—the white nymph or I am filled with Anna and my experiences or…the hole in me has been generously unemptied.

Molt 3: The birth

Today I saw the dragon-fly
Come from the wells where he did lie.
An inner impulse rent the veil
Of his old husk, from head to tail
Came out clear plates of sapphire mail.
He dried his wings: like gauze they grew;
Thro' crofts and pastures wet with dew
A living flash of light he flew.
(Tennyson, 1883, lines 8-15)[102]

Following experiences enumerated in the previous molts, such as learning to depend on, to lean on, and to trust Anna, and the subsequent opening of regressive early phases of my life, places where the early trauma took place, it seems like the poet's memory has become mine. A scaffold, the globe as a frame, has contributed to a feeling of being defined. The purpose of a working scaffold is to provide a safe working platform and access suitable for work crews to carry out their work. I feel a sheathing skin for the first time in my life: an alive scaffold enabling the work at the center to be carefully, conceptually conceived and incarnated. At the center of my being, the warring or static opposites have begun to dance and to play with each other. There is a dynamic interplay or dialogue. An amalgamation of their energies is deposited centripetally, a composite of autonomous as well as intimately alloyed energies.

---

[102] Tennyson was thinking of the suicide of his friend Arthur Henry Hallam when he wrote "The Two Voices"; is the other voice the dragonfly? The relevant portion of "The Two Voices" is located in Appendix A-3.

THE HISS OF HOPE

My early life-experiences have assumed a shape; out of the opposites of me and not-me, out of the dynamic dialogues, there is now a bilateral point in my center. It feels like Anna has become my mother, that an exchange from my biological mother to Anna has taken place inside—and outside—of me. It feels as if the others have become colors of this central point, each with its own silvery quality, each quickened through the whiteness of the "living flash of light." The others have interchanged their energies with us, and the residue is the experience of my world being held together from the inside, intrapsychically. Theoretically, the opposites have begun to flow against each other and also with each other—dynamically in relationship instead of being static and frozen. Indeed, they become self-reflexive. I do not have to be in control. I have released myself into the waters of the voyage.

Three transformational requisites for flying

"A living flash of light he flew."

In order to be able to achieve such an inner ontological shift, I want to suggest three specific relating patterns that have contributed to my transformation. First of all, Anna's uncanny ability to allow me to use her, to lean on her. Without feeling guilty, or without becoming entangled in my propensities to succeed or to fail, or without sensing an infallibility or destructibility, I have been able to use Anna in a manner appropriate for a preverbal infant (Winnicott, 1971, pp. 86-94).

This using—or leaning on—is for an adult the most difficult. It has been so for me. I've never experienced the infant's experience of omnipotence, the infant's feeling of puzzling the world together according to subjective needs only, the infant's narcissistic use of the good-enough mother. My mother's dictum, "thou shalt not be emotional," told me that I am not allowed to be myself. For me to display any intensity evokes an expression of strong disapproval on my mother's face. I feel as if I have committed a sin, that I am evil.

202

Gradually, I learn to be real *with* Anna. With feelings of guilt in the beginning, or with fear of losing her, I literally force myself to use her. Often, I think if I do not learn to do this now, I'll never have another opportunity. Anna's consistent availability and willingness to participate in this anaclitic therapy, her consciousness, and her soft and nurturing encouragement allow me to slip out of the defensive false self of this structural repetition compulsion. Together we cut through this rigid structure, a rare and unique achievement in and of itself, and especially in such a short space of time.

Secondly, Anna has been able to know, to recognize, when I am not able physically to be a hostess at dinners, or when Parkinson's would take over my body and I would not be able to continue making the gingerbread, or when we are walking, and, like a flash of lightning, Parkinson's grabs me. Anna sees these moments. Softly, she just takes over. This is often a huge relief for me. Anna's empathy has been—and is—unusual. With her preverbal infant, the good-enough mother is in a relating pattern that sets the future pattern of being with the other. It is then also the future pattern of relating between the child and her body. It becomes the foundational blueprint for the way the more mature person later relates to the world around her. Like the structure of the walls of a house determines the spaces, the patterns of relating between the mother and the infant determine her future networking in general (Neumann, 1980, p. 28).[103]

The third requisite between Anna and me that helps to cut through even the paralyzed structure of a repetition pattern is Anna's autonomy, her faith in herself, as well as her ability to be intimate. Indeed, without these defined walls to slam up against, or if she were not able to give of herself without fear of losing herself, our intimate autonomy would not have crystallized. Optimal oppositional friction,

---

[103] "In der unabgehobenen Identitaet des Kindes mit der Mutter steht die Urbeziehung gleichzeitig fuer die Beziehung zum Du, zum eigenen Koerper, zu (sich selber) und zur Welt." The primal relating pattern with the mother repeats itself in every object relationship as well as with the infant's relationship with its own body and with the world [Author's translation].

as well as soft innermost sharing, are requisites to "fly as a living flash of light." Both are as necessary as the hammer and the nail to hold a construction together. Both friction and conflict are as necessary as the harmony and the togetherness.

During this third molt, I experience quite veritably a birth. I do not fly like the dragonfly, but I do walk. All in all, it is no wonder that so many people refer to Anna as a baby whisperer.

[Her whispers] "rent the veil...
Of his [her] old husk from head to tail."

Molt 2: The split

The birth is a miscarriage. A split. A fugue phrase must have missed its turn. The composition collapses. The yawning hole screams once again.

What causes such a split in general and, more specifically, in me? And why does it insist on pulling me apart again against my conscious will? And why do the two conflicting parts always separate from each other, instead of entertaining the slightest inclination to dialogue? And to become, once again, a two and a one?

I am so glad that I know this kind of process, this voyage, is not a straight line from one oceanic wave to the next. It is not linear. Instead, I recognize that such journeys wind and twist, they soar, and they take a nosedive. I know that repetitive structures alter spirally. They seem to change, but then something happens, and you think you are right back where you were years ago. But you aren't! The rhythm is different, the momentum has transformed. Space and time have assumed other dimensions. You sense that it is not anymore just about you, but your voyage can affect the whole world. "The world hangs on a thin thread and that thread is the psyche of Man." (Jung, quoted in Evans, 1964)[104]

---

[104] "The world," said Jung, "hangs on a thin thread, and that thread is the psyche of man . . . . It is not the reality of the hydrogen bomb we must fear, but what man does with it. Suppose certain fellows in Moscow lose their nerve, then the world is in fire and flames. As never before, the world hangs on the psyche of man." Therefore, explained the wise old

With this in mind, I can regard these regressed experiences, not as nonsuccesses or failures, but rather as inevitable moments in a deeply transformative process. And I no longer not give up for my own individual sake; but there is a newly experienced sense of responsibility for a more collective, a more cultural historical dimension. I feel as if I've become enmeshed in the web of the world, caught in spun silken structures like those woven by a spider. The spider weaves its web again and again, no matter how often it is torn down. It does not give up. Is this spider-world-web an additional intricate scaffold? Does it offer me an opportunity to construct a new entity in me, or to open a third space? Or wait until these are self-quickened? Do I have to try to shed it? It feels like suddenly becoming enmeshed in an inevitable embedment of being.

The regression

Two weeks after Anna leaves, the regressive energy of anxious desperation slices through and engulfs me once again. The unfluctuating structure of the repetition compulsion claims me, opens the familiar rapacious hole of anxiety, and Thanatos' satisfied satanical smirk stops even the slightest vibration of a transformative process. Dreams disappear. Parkinson's disease becomes once again an enemy instead of a companion. Our new relationship of two dancing into a one sighs its way into its own extinction.

Once again on this voyage I am in the relentless force of the oceanic undertow—a psychic regression. I sense the strength of a devouring force sucking me down, a searing energy claiming me in its inaudible but yet muffled ultrasonic silence. Can one be buried alive in silence? I feel alone. There is no dance partner, no one with whom I can play. There is an emptiness in this nothingness.

I do tend to fly so high when a noticeable change occurs and am then catapulted into a chasm when the improvements are not all totally

---

man, the study and understanding of man's psyche is more important than ever.

sustainable. Once again, I feel lamed with the inundating feeling of giving up, the threatening negative spiral of "is all this merely an ultimate shipwreck"? Is the voyage primarily an exercise to improve my writing skills? Is Anna's and my relationship a mythopoetic miscarriage? Or is my pregnancy fated to yield one stillbirth after another? And what about the dragonfly's "flash of light"?

Dragonflies have an external skeleton, an exoskeleton. Once they leave the water, their birth process takes place on the *outside*, one could say. They are unable to mature unless they shed the old skeleton and make a new one. This shedding, or molting, can occur up to 15 times, a part of the process called *metamorphosis*. This maturation can take a whole winter to complete. The larva, or the nymph, finds a safe location away from the water; its legs stiffen and lock to the surface it is resting on. Here, the repetitive emergences commence, the fascinating unfolding of the wings being one of the last. Once the wings are full-size, the veins and vessels begin to harden in order to serve their next role as supports for the wings in flight. The dragonfly has to wait for its wings and body to dry into the hard shells that give it the rigidity needed for flight. Patience also is necessary for the emergence of the abdomen, which is divided into 10 segments containing the digestive functions as well as the sex organs. The dragonfly is prone to damage if it flies before the wings and the abdomen dry. This concluding part of the process can take several hours. The dragonfly, this amazing creature, whose life encompasses the *balancing* of water and air, is also called a *libelle*, whose etymological root means "balance fly" (Mitchell & Lasswell, 2005, p. 27).

The birth process of the libelle: The adult libelle, the mature libelle: a balance-fly. But I have lost my balance. I have once again become one-sided; I have once again regressed. My birth process feels as if it has simply stopped. The globe is still there, probably the placenta also. I know that. But I sense an immobile quality of everything…a moment of *death*? And the very familiar screams of the *hole* are again agonizingly present: anxiety, feeling half there/half here, imminent drops of tears…but mostly it is the omnipresent anxiety. And then it claims me with inaudible silence. As if I were buried in water…alive.

This anxiety feels like it has something to do with falling into this hole, with losing my identity, with disintegration. Or perhaps the anxiety fills the hole and…again has become my identity, albeit defensive. Nonetheless, whatever the task of a defense mechanism may be, my endeavor is to allow this "inner impulse (to) rent the veil/Of his old husk, from head to tail," to digest and discard this structure of repetitive compulsive defense, and to allow my "birth"—my "death"—process to finally continue. Tennyson's last verse of *In Memorium: 45* describes the immanent terror of this process:

This use may lie in blood and breath,
Which else were fruitless of their due,
Had man to learn himself anew
Beyond the second birth of Death.
(Tennyson, 1850/2014)[105]

"The birth of death"…a physical, a phenomenological experience that perhaps in fact "lies in blood and breath." And the psychological experience? Winnicott refers to a common byproduct of this two-in-one experience, of death and birth: unthinkable anxiety. He lists five differentiated aspects of this sense of annihilation: (1) going to pieces; (2) having no relation to the body; (3) having no orientation; (4) falling forever; and (5) complete isolation because of there being no means of communication (Davis & Wallbridge, 1981, p 46).

The hole's gaping emptiness once again screams without any defining structuring to sustain it, to mold the emptiness, or to lance the pain of the ragged edge of desperation. I feel an emptiness without any evidence of a collocating structure to touch and to spawn the emanation of a reflecting echo. The hole has once again assumed the characteristics of a chasm, an abyss, an emptiness, and, at the same time, an earthquake splitting, crashing, and cutting the skin holding the white globe. The globe remains uncompromisingly attached, attached by obstinate cells, coagulated blood, and the ligaments'

---

[105] The full text of "In Memorium: 45" is located in Appendix A-5.

membranous fold that supports an organ and keeps it in place. Nonetheless, the internal tearing feels like a rupture, it feels more and more like a yawning split, more and more as if it is ultimately crystallizing once again into two opposite ossified sides. These two, whose proximity once upon a time also whispers fuguelike assonant notes of no melodic harmony, now shout out Stockhausen's dissonant notes of scorn and laugh their way down into the depths where one empty, abandoned husk of the dragonfly lies. Is this what an inner impulse feels like when it "rents the veil"? Nothing new is born. Indeed, is this exposed naked emptiness the byproduct?

The vertical split

Like the exoskeleton of the dragonfly, the split frames a relating pattern (a nonrelating pattern). But instead of a structure's more familiar function, that is, to contain, to hold, to aid in constructing until such a need dissipates, the structural frame of a split serves to defensively, desperately, divide and dissociate, to divide any one into nonrelating twos, into static opposites. The inner impulse initiating the dragonfly's shedding of its exoskeleton is a split also, but not a defensive action. It is a part of an offensively dynamic process, an Eros-connected, a life-giving process rhythmically birthing and then shedding, a process of a one becoming a two, and then a one and then a two, ad infinitum…each a flowing movement mirroring and relating to each other. Each a natural symmetry, Mandelbrot's fractal of the autopoietic process of systems thinking.

Psychological splitting is not a scaffold to be shed, or an exo-skeleton to be discarded. Nor is it a structural defensive repetitive compulsion. These three are all inherently dynamic; they are part of a living, a dynamic process. But the clinical split, the frame defining the relating pattern, usually ossifies into a dead end, into a desiccated psychic movement disorder.

Pierre Janet (1849-1947) first described a psychic split. Freud further differentiated it as not derived from an innate incapacity for synthesis, but rather an inner impulse's *capacity* and proclivity to set up an impenetrable wall of protection. This pattern is initiated by the conflict of opposing mental forces, and the two ultimately freeze into a dehydrated protective division of opposite energies, opposite drives that cannot reach each other. Any spark of dynamic interchange is impeded.

In his unfinished paper of 1938, "Splitting of the Ego in the Process of Defense (*Ichspaltung*)," and later in his 1940 *Outline of Psychoanalysis*, Freud is concerned with the ego's panic about losing control, about being *ruptured* and, in a desperate act of *self-defense*, this ego causes a cleavage or division of itself: a split. The later differentiations of Otto Kernberg and Heinz Kohut in the 1970s between the vertical and the horizontal splits are concerned with preverbal trauma (vertical split) and later trauma, when the ego is at least partially formed (horizontal split) (Kohut, 1971, pp. 176-177; Kernberg, 1984).[106]

My split is vertical. Water turns to crystal. The sun becomes ice. The moon becomes silver, and time stands still. This is a preverbal split at a time when there is no self-conscious ego that could refer anything to itself, that is, reflect. Not only is the psyche open to the world, it is identical with and undifferentiated from the world; it knows itself as world and in the world and experiences itself as a world becoming, its own images as the starry heavens, and its own contents as the world-creating gods (Neumann, 1995, p 60).

This experience of omnipotence is a defensive structure of the mind to ensure its split-off opposite of devaluation will remain statically in place. Both omnipotence and devaluation are subjectively experienced and objectively projected. There is no third space offering a potential place of communication, or the tremor of an emotion evoking oppositional curiosity. Or the serenity of a center force. If the two sides of the split were to dynamically dialogue, they would both fold into each other and rupture the desperate defensive organizational pattern. The poet prompts once again:

---

[106] Horizontal split: Traumatic event(s) occurs after ego nuclei have come together and partial identity has been formed. Dull throbs are felt, depression, fear. Vertical split occurs before ego nuclei have come together. A mere hint of identity. Hardly anything is felt except disintegration anxiety. A horizontal split is a break between the ego and the unconscious; the vertical split is an ego break. See added papers on vertical split in Molt 2.

"Turning and turning in the widening gyre
…things fall apart; the centre cannot hold…"
(Yeats, 1921/1969)[107]

A further dissociation or even a disintegration of the personality is the more common response to the fear of losing cohesion.[108]

If the mother does not gaze into the infant's eyes with connection, the preverbal infant feels catapulted out of the mother's environment: There is no experience of being contained by the mother. When the mother's eyes do not mirror her, the infant does not find herself, either physically nor psychically. The infant experiences herself as a nothing, a nonentity. In the first three months, there is but little ego to fill the emptiness of the nonconnecting relating pattern between the mother and the baby. The preverbal infant's psyche splits. It creates a *false self* that protects the true self by the isolation of the latter from reality. The interpersonal splitting of the mother and the baby reflects itself in the subsequent internal or intrapsychic split of the infant.

Ironically, this split itself continues to nurture the separateness. The nonmeeting of the infant's eyes with the mother's mirrors the infant as a nothing. This feeling of being nonexistent becomes one of the repetition compulsive endeavors of the child throughout her life. Without some kind of therapeutic intervention, this person will be impelled to create situation after situation in which she will not be seen. She does not dare to be "discovered."

---

[107] The full text of Yeat's poem "The Second Coming" is located in Appendix A-8.

[108] For those interested in attachment theories: Melanie Klein, Anna Freud and their successors, Wilfred Bion, and D.W. Winnicott, splitting is a defensive dissociation and distortion in the mother and the baby's environment.
For further reading on attachment theories see the following: Freud, A. and Burlingham, D. (1944). Infants without families. New York: International Universities. Klein, M. (1946). The early development of the conscience in the child. In M. Klein Contributions to psycho-analysis 1921-1945 (pp. 282-310). London: Hogarth. Bion, W. (1984). Learning from experience. London: Karnic/Maresfield Reprints. Guntrip. H. Psychoanalytic theory, therapy and the self. New York: Basic. Neumann, E. (1976). The child. New York: Harper Colophon. Winnicott, D. W. (1949). Mind and its relations to the psyche-soma. In Paediatrics to Psychoanalysis (pp. 243-254). New York: Basic. Winnicott, D. W. (1965). The maturation processes and the facilitating environment. London: Hogarth. Winnicott, D. W. (1971). Playing and reality. London: Tavistock. An excellent more recent publication summarizing attachment theory is: Wallib, D. J. (2015). Attachment in psychotherapy. New York: Guilford.

Vertically split, a person can feel like an abandoned, desperate child on Monday. On Tuesday, she is confident and powerful in her new job as CEO of a successful business organization. On Wednesday, she has pain in her back and can barely walk upright, or a migraine that forces her to remain at home in bed. On Thursday, she is madly in love, and on Friday, she wonders what she ever saw in the man. On the weekend, she is terrified to be alone, so she makes one date after another, and by Sunday evening she is totally exhausted.

The structure is fragmentation. There is no centripetal force holding the pieces together. The holding force, the inner residue of the introjected good-enough mother, is nonexistent. There is no center; there is no core whose inner impetus sheds the exoskeleton of the dragonfly. There is no bilateral point to coordinate Thanatos and Eros and thereby to know when to rupture the structure of her defensive repetition compulsion. And to learn myself (herself) anew.

This skeletal structural provision becomes the ossified repetition compulsion, which Freud associates with the death instinct. How can I spark an inner impulse to switch off the compulsive allure of Thanatos, to once again constellate Eros, to dynamically reenter into the life-bestowing process Anna and I once had experienced? How can I shed this regressive husk in order to molt and emerge like the dragonfly "beyond the second birth of Death"?

Is there a truth to the new insight in chaos theory that even "the endpoint of chaos has structure at a global level and that out of it emerges yet another order"? (Robertson, 2009, p. 6) Can chaos inhere a potential quickening and "shed the split"? Like the dragonfly nymph's process of shedding each exoskeleton? Perhaps like Jung's idea that "only he remains vitally alive who is ready to die with life," Goethe's "die and become" (*stirb und werde*), or Tennyson's "beyond the second birth of Death" (Jung, CW 8, 1960/1981, para. 800).[109]

---

[109] Jung's description emphasizes the ego's "Death," the ego's relinquishing its power to the Self. And Goethe's last verse of Selige Sehnsucht: "Und so lang du das nicht hast,/ Dieses: Stirb und Werde!/ Bist du nur ein trueber Gast auf der dunklen Erde." As long as you do not have this, /This: to die and to be born again/ you remain but a hollow guest on this dark earth. [Author's translation.]

Each of these envisions a two-in-one world, a notion of dynamic dialectic opposites rather than static divided polarities, a concept scientifically valid as well as immanently alchemical. A pattern of relating. Can a death initiate a birth, can destruction open to creativity, can man "learn himself anew," and can I envision myself as a two in one and render my static split dynamic through a relating pattern? Can an old protective repetition compulsion die into a second birth? Can a chasm protect and then reveal a valley canyon of fecund curiosity that doesn't "unripen to a bud," as Winnicot wrote, but also opens to Tennyson's "crofts and pastures wet with dew"?

Isaac Newton, the scientific alchemist

Instead of dualistic opposition, a split between two, the renowned scientist Isaac Newton envisions a two birthing itself out of a one, then infusing each other, impregnating each other. He personifies the dynamism as well as the veracity inevitable in this third-space perspective.

Standing in this third space between alchemy and science, at that pivot point between the 17th and 18th centuries, Isaac Newton the alchemist is at the same time one of the most important persons in the history of science. Isaac Newton, who changes the world forever with his scientific discoveries, also translates *The Emerald Tablet of Hermes Trismegistus* from the Latin. Isaac Newton, who sees the world of science with its empirical absolutes, also knows (*kennen*) the deeper world revealed by alchemy as unalterable constituent parts of an intimate autonomy, a two-in-one inevitability. Isaac Newton integrates and balances alchemy of the Middle Ages, the power or the process that changes, that transforms "from an inner impulse" in mysterious ways, with his science space of empirical data.

Science (from Latin *scientia*, meaning "knowledge") is a quantitative, systematic process of gathering knowledge. Using exclusively empirical facts, albeit sometimes intangible, scientists explain something as yet unknown as something to be disovered in the near future. The quality of presence is not relevant. Rationality is the key. One could be inclined to view alchemy and science as irreconcilable opposites, as incommensurable. Newton refutes this all-or-nothing dualistic manner of thinking. Instead of splitting them, he reconciles the two into one. Along with the other 14 points of the alchemical *Emerald Tablet*, Newton translates the second item, a line that refutes a split existence and reiterates the illusion of separation. This second point also reflects the dragonfly's transmutation. The dragonfly frees itself from the husk of structural incarceration, rebroadcasts and reimages its existence as the *balance fly*, as a gradual two in one. The second line of the *Emerald Tablet*, this significant descriptive dialectical dynamic, reads: "That which is below is like that which is above & that which is above is like that which is below to do ye miracles of *One* only thing" (Robertson, 2009, p. 22).

It does help to remind myself of the alchemical dictum: Life is a boomerang swinging from *separatio* to *coagulatio*, back and forth and forth and back, as well as feeling the placenta and its etymological root and the ancient rhythm of bread, taking apart and putting back together of the dough over and over, separating parts of the dough that are close together and bringing together other parts that are widely separated. "…. only separated things can unite, the alchemist reminds us." (Edinger, 1995, p. 280) Also, I am able still to feel the faint stirring of the dragonfly nymph. If I had not been able to repeat these ancient mantras, if I had not known a possibility of this regression potentially being a husk to shed, or a repetition compulsion to reinvent, rather than an imprisoning impregnable wall, and—perhaps most importantly—if I had not known of the strength of an inner impulse, of giving up ego control to some other source, I could have been too discomposed and too discouraged to continue the voyage.

If I had not experienced the relating pattern of an intimate autonomy with Anna, as well as with such inner figures as the pitbull and the kittens, I would not have had a new structure, a firm yet moving scaffold to hang on to.

An additional help is remembering dream contents that accompanied me while Anna was still here.[110] I attempt to soak in these

---

[110] Some dreams from September 17, 2013, to October 20, 2013:

images, to release myself to the dragonfly, to not think but to experience myself as the object of a thought rather than the subject. I let the mantras flow; I try to *not try*. I wait until the pitbull rages and the various kittens enter into an intimately autonomous relating pattern with each other and with me.

Eventually, I note slight faint—but factual—stirrings of silent *chi* energy waking up my core. It is physical. It is like Billy Elliot's finely attuned stretch and whirl in the air, when the body takes over and hones a final secret twist into eternity. My leap is also an internal physical and psychic dynamic. Eventually, I do shed a skeletal husk, an aged structure of "protector turned perpetrator" (Kalsched, 1996).

The process continues. My regression has opened to "beyond the birth of death." Thoughts yield once again to feelings; Thanatos opens to Eros, death bows once again to life.

There remains but one conceived notion to elucidate further. As my father has reiterated about architectural design, the structure yields to the space. In our case, the design of anaclitic therapy yields to a space where a good-enough mother can be introjected, where an intimacy and vulnerability reflective of the first months of life can be experienced and assumed. This rerun of a preverbal space enables an intimate autonomous relating pattern to blossom, thereby negating to a great degree the tendency to "unripen into a bud." Potentially, anaclitic therapy structures a space that offers the freedom to learn to fall apart,

---

I would take glass things in my hand and somehow they would break. These glass things were antique and beautiful. They reminded me of the wings of the dragonfly. The color white: "Eins und Alles," all colors, all shades of colors and simultaneously one color. The colors become dynamic with light "breaking" through white.

There was a little girl and her parents. They all had dark hair. The parents were laughing and were full of joy; the girl also. Then the little girl came up to a kind of interface between her and me, she stood there and looked into my eyes intensely. Her eyes again were the eyes of the blind kitten. She looked straight at me. I felt a connection, no anxiety, just connection.

I was with two other women who were in a loving lesbian relationship. I wanted to find a silver suit, skin tight—sort of like skiers wear. We were in a lift going up to the thirteenth floor to find this suit. One wall was a mirror. A woman stood in front of this mirror, she was dark like the child before with the eyes, she look penetratingly at me and said twice: "You know."

Dream of a small furry fetus-type creature and I felt a powerful love for it. I kept stroking, caressing it, and holding it softly.

to surrender ego strength, without the fear of losing oneself and its corresponding capacity and propensity to relate with the openness and the privilege of vulnerability.

Figure: Horizontal and Vertical Split

These drawings are how I visualize the horizontal and vertical splits conceived by Heinz Kohut and Otto Kernberg (see footnote 601).

With a HORIZONTAL SPLIT, traumatic events occur *after* ego nuclei have come together. This consolidation leads to a partial identity core. With this partial integration the ego has enough strength to push the 'unwanted' personality traits into the unconscious and can try to ignore or to forget them. 'She' feels nonetheless dull throbs, depression and fear. The defense mechanisms often employed are rationalization, intellectualization, workaholism, and repression.

With a VERTICAL SPLIT, traumatic events occur *before* ego nuclei have come together. This leads to an unconsolidated identity. The psyche splits the ego to avoid the pain of disintegration anxiety. 'She' is one person on Monday, on Tuesday she identifies with someone else, and so on throughout the week. She feels hardly anything except disintegration anxiety. Further defense mechanisms can be idealization, projective identification, devaluation and omnipotence, and reaction formation.

Molt 1: Anaclitic therapy

Rene Spitz's 1946 introduction of the concept of anaclitic depression describes a specific kind of suffering present in young children that is caused by maternal deprivation. Spitz coined the word, *anaclitic* (leaning upon), since these children had no one to lean on—to use—for the nurturance they required. The concept of anaclitic therapy first becomes part of the treatments in psychiatry and psychoanalysis. For this kind of therapy to be effective, the patient returns to the space of the trauma. It is in this space of regression that reorganization is possible.

Regression revisited

Regression is a term first introduced by Freud in *The Interpretation of Dreams* (1900) and becomes a key concept in psychoanalysis in the mid-20th century. Beginning in the 1950s, it is a central factor in analytic and psychiatric anaclitic therapies. The anaclitic *leaning on*, a natural relating pattern for an infant, is more difficult for an adult. This assumption leads to the hypothesis that a regressed adult is more likely to lean, more likely to allow herself to become dependent on the caregiver. In psychiatric clinics it soon becomes normal to induce a regression by such violating, invasive methods as electroconvulsive therapy (ECT). Drugs (including psychedelic drugs), sleep deprivation, and even isolation become common and accepted means to manipulate regression. "Indeed the systematic disregard for the patient's expressed wishes is highlighted in the publications on this form of treatment." (Raz, 2010, p. 56)

    During and after a regressive phase in anaclitic therapy, the patient is seen by the psychotherapist three or four times daily, including the weekends. For many anaclitic therapists, as well as for psychoanalysts, regression remains a key experience in an anaclitic therapy or analysis in general; for others, it becomes gradually more and more irrelevant. As British analyst Wilford Bion's often-cited aphorism highlights:

"Winnicott says patients need to regress; Melanie Klein says they must not regress; I say they *are* regressed." (Bion, 1992, p. 166)

For Anna and me, regression assumes the role endemic to psychoanalysis, as we both know it from Germany. An intimate relationship in the analysis, a relationship mirroring more of the healthy close attachment between the mother and infant, is what we experience as the spark to trigger a regression, a return to a former or less developed state, where one can dismember and then remember. With the firm holding of anaclitic therapy's scaffold, ego control can be at least partially surrendered in an open space of potential reorganization. A reconstruction of an autonomous personality that is open to intimacy, a relating pattern whose sine qua non is a dynamic flow, reflects the "road traveled" to get there. The trajectory has been the structure of a two-in-one relating pattern rather than the more clinically practiced hierarchical and dualistic perpetrator/victim dynamic, the structure set up in the psychiatric use of electric shock.

In our experience, a regression is most often attainable if the interpersonal relating pattern between the two—between Anna and me—becomes close enough, if sufficient containment, if moments—or even seconds—of a oneness are felt. In this new space of relative safety, defense mechanisms begin to dissolve. Catapulted then back into the space of the original trauma, into the feelings, the emotions, and the physical memories, which have been lost with the vertical split, our regressive space allows an encounter with all these previously unconscious entities. But this time with different environmental factors. It is at these moments that an analytic anaclitic therapeutic relationship can contribute to a reformation, to a suspension—perhaps even to a shattering—of the incarcerating walls of the defensive repetition compulsions. Indeed, it is one of Freud's most important discoveries. If the impact of the inundating tensions does not submerge the present ego, if their reintroduction does not invoke a repetition of the anxiety splitting the newborn's tiny ego, if the intimate autonomous relationship of Anna and me can reflect onto and into this regressed space, then the regressive space opens to reorganization, to feelings and experiences both terrifying and soaring with joy.

Once again, I experience being the newly born infant on the weighing scale in a room all by myself. But this time when I cry or when I scream, Anna is there. She seems to take over and manage the regression, filling the space with softness, with care, and in whose eyes I see myself loved and cherished. She becomes the good-enough mother I can lean on. Gradually, the abyss due to the vertical split fills with an entity mirroring the awareness that Anna and I, that our relating patterns, are the central centripetal force holding everything together. Gradually, I get to know this quality of presence even without Anna being physically present. Gradually, the third space is constellated, harboring, holding, and inhering the optimal oppositional friction necessary for a balanced, liquid flow of energy. This one in two contains intimately at the same time that it opens up to—and quickens—autonomy. Gradually, the dialectical ingenuity governs the relating pattern between this center and me, as well as the relating pattern between Anna and me, and gradually assumes the structures of an intimate autonomy.

The strength and warranty of this center is the byproduct of Anna's initial holding of my loose trembling until I can *swallow*—or introject, digest, and sustain—the intensity of her oscillating vibrations as well as my own. First, I have to become acquainted with the feelings and vibratory fluctuations present in Anna, and then, secondly, I need to become familiar with the shared innuendoes in our pattern of relating. And I have to learn to trust them. If I am unable to rely on Anna and an *us*, I can probably not learn to rely on myself and will trust the old, known, defensive vertical split once again.

My regression is not induced through invasive tactics; my regression has been a byproduct of the introjection (my "eating and digesting") of Anna and of her good-enough-mother nurturing. When this incorporation takes place, the moment I eat or interiorize or introject the experience of Anna and her manner of caring for me, my defenses can begin to melt like Galatea, like "wax under the sun." My ego, my willpower, my need to control Anna, my inclination to fight Parkinson's disease, my usual practice of commanding my body, seem to dissipate into thin air. Instead of the practice of defensive dualistic competition and mastery, I begin to be able to survive in a relationship with the other as object and as subject; that is, with me directing Parkinson's and with the feeling that today Parkinson's has the upper hand.

The fragmentation of the repetition compulsion is the most difficult moment in analysis and the most necessary. It is the intra-psychic mirrored moment transferring the outside to the inside: the interpersonal to the intrapsychic. A new relating pattern. A new world. I hear the echo of our interpersonal holding patterns resounding in me, and I can know the reverberations of the abyss being filled with the energized melodies quickening more and more notes of a new firm-ness, solidity, and a strength hitherto unknown. I can know for the first time the rhythm and the sounds of an internal and an external relating pattern, a fugue of contrapuntal distance and closeness, an intimate autonomy instead of the terror of the vacuous pit of anxiety and emptiness.

The third space revisited

There are different sources vibrating, reverberating, and relating simultaneously: the two centers of Anna and of me; and a third space where the intersecting force of the intimate autonomy holds firmly the two (or the three or more) in the one. Converging realities, merging worlds.

Our anaclitic therapy takes place in this third space where different worlds gather, where opposite worlds can convene, clash, and converse. A center, a core, gradually unfolds holding these worlds together, or a bilateral point assumes form and introduces yet additional—and probably a more desperate and a more demanding—attunement. Worlds of imagination, of mytho-poetics and mysticism, worlds of psychic and physical realities, and the worlds of culture, of science, of power, and of passion contend and concur. Hovering in the ever-increasing vibration emanating from the center, the separation, the competition, the animosity among the many worlds can often gradually fine-tune to one song, one hymn, while at the same time each world can retain its own unique autonomy. The holding at the center allows a centripetal contrapuntal composition of many voices. A unified duality (*geeinte Zweinatur*) (Goethe, 1806/1992, line 11962), a unified multiplicity, a pattern's fugue of relationship.

The third space

The third space is not a literal, concrete place. It is not Winnicott's transitional space, nor is it Jung's transcendent function. It is more like Hegel's synthesis: the culmination of the duality of *thesis and antithesis* and the emergence of yet another round of relationship. Or another fractal of the form of a relating pattern. Hegel calls it "the *dialectical* moment in thought, the fact that, when thought properly, the 'initial universal determines itself out of itself to be the *other of itself*" (Houlgate, 1991, p. 38). It is energy. It is process. It begins to unfold as soon as the touch between the two is experienced, and it evaporates when this relating pattern of the two in one is withdrawn. It is a rhythm. It is the dancing-stillness space of paradox. And beyond. An earthed hovering. Conceptually, this third space has the purity of a geometrical form, the beauty and the mystery of an alchemical vase, or the quality of the enfolding arms of a good-enough mother. A welcoming space, an enveloping space, a holding and sustaining space to drink from. A space where the infant on the weighing scale is waiting to be discovered, to be seen, and to be loved. And then a space to leave. But to return again and again, rhythmically, until it becomes a part of you, until it incarnates in you. For the rest of your life and perhaps even at the moment of your death—you can return when you so desire. And you can drink. Or you can dance to ancient fugues. This space is a nourishing nothingness that fills and replenishes you with everything, a paradoxical space of creative, transforming emptiness. It is a place, however, that demands courage and curiosity to enter. You often have to leap.

I just thought of all the worlds, of all the forces involved in the intersubjectivity of an anaclitic process: Anna's ego, Anna's inner center, my ego, my center…or lack thereof. Perhaps one could say my abyss. And the process itself generates its own defensive as well as offensive energies. We can benefit from such a conductor as the recently deceased Claudio Abbado, who claimed that there is a certain sound to snow, a sound he can hear when the snowflakes fall. The sound is a particular note of silence that then fades away like a breath. He had learned that skill from his maternal grandfather, an expert in ancient languages. Abbado does not dominate the music he directs but is its servant. Orchestra members under his baton become so attuned to each other while at the same time listening for snowflakes in their own music that—like for Abbado—music becomes a thing of magic, created, vanishing, then waiting to be created again. A third space. His obituary notes that when half of Abbado's digestive system was removed in 2000 because of cancer, Abbado joked that he could now hear from inside his body, a gaunt and sounding shell. His concerts became more illuminating, more infused with love, as if each note were found afresh (Claudio Abbado, obituary, 2014).

In an attempt to clarify, to quicken, to breathe life into the words *anaclitic therapy* as well as into the paradoxical nature of this relationship fugue, Anna and I have discussed our experience up until now and have documented some of our thoughts and our observations:

A personal account of anaclitic therapy

Meredith (M): First of all, I would like to talk about our relationship with each other before concentrating more on each one of us individually. It is perhaps relevant to keep in mind the term coined as appropriately descriptive for our work together: It has been a process, *a relating pattern of an intimate autonomy.*

So, Anna, if you look at our process up until now, what do you consider to be the central features?

Anna (A): For me, an attitude of openness and curiosity are cornerstone characteristics of anaclitic therapy, of our process unfolding into a balanced relationship of an intimate yet autonomous relating pattern. Contributing to the actual timing of our endeavor is, of course, the often-frightening violence of your Parkinson's disease and your anxiety. We have been—and still are—open to what we still do not know. We have been observant—and remain observant—regarding beneficial as well as potentially more negative results of our work.

M: Yes, I agree. A kind of pitbull determination reflective of Parkinson's tenacity, an open and receptive attitude as well as a curious posture and a kittenlike instinctual autonomy are requisites for any process and especially for one as intimate, one that demands such constant physical and psychological attending as ours. Sometimes it feels like the swift darting of the dragonfly, and, at other times, the requisite is the stillness of the poet's dance (Eliot, 1943).[111]

Anna, would you please talk a little about our individual personalities, as well as certain relational patterns, which have contributed to our decision to undertake this relatively unknown and certainly challenging anaclitic process?

A: *Ja, gerne.* For me, the most important relational quality is our mutual respect, our knowing that we can rely on the other, a byproduct of my long analysis with you in Frankfurt. It was such an awe-inspiring and new experience for me, an experience that changed me at my deepest core and reshaped my whole life.

In addition, my knowledge gained from many professional years as a pediatric nurse and, more recently, the years working as a psychiatric nurse, and as a baby whisperer, certainly contribute to our process. Due to these experiences, I recognize the central significance of emphasizing both the physical and the psychological states of the

---

[111] "...except for the still point/there is no dance/And there is only the dance." The full text of "Burnt Norton II" is located in Appendix A-1.

patient. A quantitative, a diagnostic approach is not enough. I have found that much has to be perceived intuitively; I have to feel things, to sense things. In order for this to be possible, a physical proximity is advantageous. I must be able to hold, to lift up, and to physically take care of a patient. For example, during these grueling nights with you, Meredith, and your Parkinson's disease.

M. Yes, Anna. Your manner of taking care of me when I am unable to even move gives me a sense of a physical containment hitherto unknown. This shift from needing subjective control to experiencing and yielding to moments of objective containment is central for me. I can imagine that as a result of your ability to accommodate, to persistently be there to hold me, something has shifted inside me, and I experience more and more being able to integrate or to consolidate my own anxiety. This new center that I've already mentioned, reflects our outside relating and holds me together now on the inside. The inside becomes the outside: a movement back and forth and forth and back. A dynamic dialectical communication. And the fierce anxiety often dissolves "in its own water."

It is perhaps also significant to mention that in the beginning of our anaclitic process, I was unable to allow you to hold my hand when I was caught by Parkinson's. In this situation, I always feel I had to be alone to cope with the intensity of Parkinson's violent and overwhelming imprisonment. Your attempt to come into this space threatened my [ego] control. Now I welcome your physical touch during these attacks. And once again, your outside containment has wandered inside me, and I experience now someone or something firmly holding me from the inside out. Hmm, sort of like the gingerbread being flipped over.

In addition to your ability to so often be present to my physical and my emotional needs, to empathize, I've noted you *feeling into* your own physical and emotional waves of potential flooding. Both of these skills—learned later or perhaps at a mother's breast—are quite foreign to me. The most profound image for me of your tending to and caring for yourself is of you sitting for hours in the brown chair in the living room with Howdy —the neighborhood cat—on your lap. You just sit there calmly for hours. Amazing! You're just staring into space. *Glotzen*, you call it. You deem these moments as your most creative times. In this stillness, there is the dance. For you, these are the moments of conscious regression, of digestion, of introjection, and integration.

I have yet another question for you, Anna. We have noted how I have changed up until now, but are you aware of any changes, any different "lenses" you might have now? What I mean is: Do you see things differently now? In an anaclitic process, where leaning on is the etymological, the root meaning, of the word *anaclitic*, it is difficult to imagine that only one leans on the other. Both lean, so to speak. It simply would not work if only one of us was the wise shamanistic leader and was always right when in conflict. Or that only one of us gives and the other takes. The pattern of the good-enough mother is our structural guide, but for two adults the content has to be another. Perhaps one could describe it as two aligned and melodiously intersecting fugue phrases.

A: Yes, definitely, I have changed also. I recognize that my inner borders have been stretched. Often, I think: *ach Ich kann nicht mehr* (everything is too much!), both physically and psychically! I just can't stand anymore of this. Especially at night, of course. But now I seem to sail through such stresses. And to reply to your second point: When I am being a baby whisperer to a newborn infant who has not been traumatized, I assume that it *eats* what I have to offer. I am *right*, I manage, and I am not concerned with myself changing. With an infant who has been injured either psychically or physically it is another matter. I then have to be open to any sudden dramatic change, to be conscious of the fact that a false interpretation or any impulsive, aggressive, or non-connected reaction could thwart any attempt to contribute to the infant's healing. I have to be open and willing to alter opinions or even to be changed at a core level.

With an infant it is one thing; with an adult it is another. And with you, Meredith, it is often so difficult for me because I can feel, I can intuit your behavior, but your actions are sometimes so hard to understand. Even now, after all the nights, all the days and hours I have put so much effort into, you still *run* away from me too often. It feels like a sheet of ice has been put between us. I cannot reach you. Admittedly, it happens less and less, but—*ach!*— it is so frustrating! This is a good example of a situation in which I have to remain open, I have to be willing to experience something new; otherwise, our process would just stop. I have to lean on you in such cases in order to allow the process to flow; that is, I have to lean on you and be receptive, I have to listen, I have to be willing to expect something coming from you, something which could help me figure out why you do this. If I were to just remain with my own feelings, if I were to remain merely concerned with myself, I would just give up, I would be totally frustrated. And I would probably assume your guilt—so to speak. I would think that we had failed and that it was all your fault.

M: *Ja*, Anna. I can really understand what you are saying. It makes me remember that terrible night when we both had slept but little. I constantly woke you up to help me to the bathroom, where I have organized a kind of gymnastic setup. I sit there and move and stretch my legs until I am free. Free means that I can walk and move where and when I want. This stretching process can take over an hour, but the experience of being free is golden. My strong will and my otherwise healthy body most often behave the way I want, and I am successful. Sometimes, however, I fail. Either I haven't slept enough, or eaten enough or…hmm, just the fact that I still attempt to assume—after all this time—a cause-and-effect edifice I can count on exemplifies my desperate need to control.

But on this night for some unknown reason, my ego just deflates. I simply have no strength, no will. I have to call you and wake you up once again. You come. I cannot sense any frustration, any anger. You do look exhausted but otherwise you are there. You are still there for me. All of a sudden, something clicks in me. It is as if a long searched-for puzzle piece had been found. Suddenly, I get it: Your ceaseless and—for the most part—calm or at the least with humor—manner of staying with me no matter what, your own inner reflection of *remaining* with yourself no matter what, allows me, indeed thrusts me, into an unfamiliar terrifying space of no control. In this space of unthinkable anxiety, I have always been totally alone. In fact, caught in this repetition compulsion, I realize that I have always erected an ice wall around me to assure my aloneness, which protects my control. I remember then always running away from my mother, instead of toward her. In the opposite direction of my actual need. Of course, then, Anna, I run away from you or I put a sheet of ice between us. Being alone and invisible affords me security and protection. Only then do I feel safe. If I had not experienced your persistent holding, I probably could not have remembered this behavior pattern.

A: And I understand on a deeper level now why my giving so much does not bind you to me exclusively, but rather, it evokes your old pattern of running away. It is so important to see now and to emphasize that only giving in and of itself is not necessarily a healing action. In fact, this *Mutter* Teresa syndrome can be potentially dangerous, both for the giver and for the taker. It can even unfold into the *identification with the aggressor* switch.

For our respective abilities to not get stuck in a difficult situation is a prerequisite to be able to enter into such a process of attachment, or —what do we call it? A relationship based on an intimate autonomy. And more specifically, the longer we are together, the closer—or more intimate—we become, the more autonomous I feel. It's ironic. Or perhaps you would claim it is paradoxical.

M: Yes, I am glad that you brought these words up again: *intimate*, *autonomous*, and even *paradox*. One could regard an intimate autonomy as oppositional, and then it would be a pattern of relating where each opposite could cancel the other one out. And perhaps it does present such a possibility if one does gets stuck in one opposite or the other. Neither one of us seems to be inclined to have to remain in such a glue, to have to get stuck in such an "I am right" dualistic power battle. Or, for that matter, to remain in a relating pattern that is too close or too distant.

But let's look at this point more closely. For me, it is the sine qua non of our work together. Intimacy implies a close—almost an adjacent—adjoining; whereas autonomy suggests a more distant relating. I can foresee the question: Can there be such a relating pattern of this nature, is it really possible to interact in a space harboring such opposing energies?

Actually, these do not have to be oppositional; instead, they constitute a paradox, a positioning of words and their meaning that sparks conflict and movement that deems dialectic inevitable. The philosopher writes:

> But one must not think ill of the paradox, for the paradox is the passion of thought, and the thinker without the paradox is like the lover without passion: a mediocre fellow. ... This, then, is the ultimate paradox of thought: to want to discover something that thought itself cannot think (Kierkegaard, 1844, p. 37).

Thinking, according to Hannah Arendt, is the conversation between the *me* and the *not-me* (Arendt, 1978).[112]

A result of such a conversation can perhaps be the experience of a pattern, a structure that *thought cannot think*. But there is, nonetheless, a combination in the form of a dynamic interchange. And the trajectory does not have to be the subjective process of thinking or the more objective positioning of being thought. Of course, I assume dynamic rather than static energy of optimal oppositional friction; that is, there is a flowing rather than a frozen movement to the whole subject/object encounter. There is a dialectic between the two, a space where the two can flow into a one and then out again. Or, for that matter, between any two there can be a path to a one through dialogue, or dialectic, or play, or dance. And there is a space for these *touching* and these *withdrawal* movements: a third space between and not-between.

---

[112] Hannah Arendt's fame stems to some extent from her words: "the banality of evil." She wrote them in her book Eichmann in Jerusalem: A Report on the Banality of Evil. She reported on the trial for The New Yorker; her first report was published in the February 16, 1963, issue. In her later book, The Life of the Mind (1978), she focuses mainly on the notion of thinking as a solitary dialogue between Me and Myself.

Anna, are there any other aspects of our anaclitic process which you deem worthy of attention?

A: Yes, now that you mention it. I have noticed that neither competition nor envy seems to play a role between us. Nor do we get stuck in dualistic power games. I am conscious of the fact that you could use Parkinson's to wield power over me and everybody else. But you don't. You seldom complain. You don't seem to experience yourself as defenseless or impotent. You aren't, hmmm, always narcissistic—or perhaps I should say—you are not overly narcissistic.

M: I must interrupt and suggest that positive narcissism can be instrumental in helping me deal with such a violent and devouring disease such as Parkinson's. In addition, I want to talk more about narcissism. I will get back to it. But Anna, I would not dare to wield Parkinson's as a power tool while relating with you. You would see through that in a second. And I would hope by now, that even I could see through it! So please continue…

A: I am interested in what you want to say regarding narcissism, but first I would like to finish my thoughts regarding individual personality traits that could contribute to an anaclitic process. One thing about me that certainly contributes is that, instead of becoming stuck in my frustration and feelings of impotence because you do not change any faster, I can note it and then tell myself to let the process itself take over instead of my exerting power over the therapy. In order to be able to do this, I recognize the inner containment I gained in my work with you in Frankfurt. I can now contain intense feelings and emotions, instead of feeling at their mercy.

M: Thank you, Anna. Such summaries can help to make difficult concepts and ideas more clearly comprehensible. Often, in addition, they elicit relevant thoughts otherwise lost or even questions otherwise forgotten. Illustrations can also contribute to a better understanding.

Part Three

Anecdotes from our anaclitic therapy

1. We both enjoy a sense of humor, which includes such structural, or linguistic, patterns of teasing each other, of laughing at one another without feeling insulted or criticized, without becoming angry or annoyed. For example, Anna tells the following anecdote: "Even though I have emphasized the necessity to wear rubber boots in such a winter climate as Edmonton, when you in the depth of winter still insist on wearing high heels outside on the icy streets and you stumble, do not think I will not grin and say *PG* [*Pech gehabt*—tough luck]." With contagious humor we laugh and tease each other. Neither one of us is insulted or feels belittled. Anna continues to implore me to put appropriate shoes on, and I continue to wear high heels.

2. Another example of attachment in an intimate autonomy that we have observed is that neither of us seems to be inclined to get stuck in a dualistic power battle. I find that one of the most transparent examples is our driving together in a car. I can't drive anymore due to Parkinson's disease, so Anna always drives. Since she is used to driving in Germany, she drives especially fast, noticeably aggressive. (Perhaps one could also say *self-assertive*.) She does not slow down long before a stop sign or a red light, or for that matter, when a car flashes red brake lights in front of her. Instead, she races up to where she is forced to stop or bang into the car ahead. Only then does she put on the brakes. In the meantime, I am sitting in the passenger seat groaning and putting my feet on imaginary brakes as well as yelling, "Stop!" every now and then. This has been going on for some time now, yet neither has changed in any manner whatsoever: Anna still drives like a German, and I still yell and groan and brake. At the most, we laugh.

This is a prime example of intimate autonomy at work. And, once again, I remember the words of Irigaray (2002, pp. 9-10):

> from this interaction between the subjective and the objective of two worlds, a third arises of which the expanse is generated thanks to the withdrawal imposed by difference.

… Thus never a completeness of the One, but constitution of Two worlds open and in relation with one another, and which give birth to a third world as work in common and space-time to be shared. The intimacy of being autonomously true to oneself while granting the other a mirrored self-intimacy and autonomy awakens this third space—an inevitable—and perhaps a necessary piece of anaclitic therapy.

3. Yet an additional example of a healthy attachment as part of an anaclitic process is that I now know that I can use Anna. I have interiorized this reaction or action. I do not even question it. I just do it. Or I do not use her. But now I can decide, because I know what it feels like. And I can *feel into* her; I know for the most part when not to use her.

A dream

I dream about a house that collapses. In the house with me is my architect father. After we work our way out of this slow organic destruction into the fresh green trees and fragrance of the spring flowers outside, he insists on returning to view the architectural engineering and to observe the demise of the structural connections and its collapse. This back and forth and forth and back went on for some time. And then as if "an inner impulse rent the veil/of his old husk from head to tail," the house finally gasps and becomes part of the dust on which it had been standing. My father shows no interest in examining connections anymore. We are free to attend to other matters.

Am I shredding a house husk? In dreams, a house is most often a symbol of the dreamer herself. In this dream it feels as if I am shedding an (dragonfly) exoskeleton as part of my metamorphoses. Am I opening on the inside to allow a new inner structure to evolve? It takes a long time for the abdomen of the dragonfly to be formed. Perhaps my digestive system is being restructured. I listen. I observe. Back and forth and forth and back.

Final Molt: The dance of colors

My voyage with Parkinson's has been an odyssey with a mediator, a guide, and a mother. Anna and our third-space processing have transported me out of the water and onto firm land. I want to remind us once again of Ahab's relating pattern with the White Whale. It is one of identification, retribution, and revenge. Our relating pattern has been one of a conscious intimate autonomy rather than the unconscious dualistic power battle Melville depicts between Ahab and the whale. Their relating pattern reflects retribution and revenge, projective identification, and separation. Moby Dick has taken Ahab's leg. Ahab's "fiery hunt" centers on a mirrored wounding of the whale. Their demise—like their relationship—is not a dynamic two in a one. Melville describes it as one hungry vortex of black drops of oceanic water that devours Ahab and threatens Ishmael. What happens to the white whale, Melville leaves open.

"But pull on! Aye, all alive, now——we near him." Ahab was fairly within the smoky mountain mist, which thrown off from the whale's spout, curled.… [Ahab] darted his fierce iron, and his far greater curse into the hated whale, "He turns to meet us!… Oh…for one red cherry ere we die! … Towards thee I roll, thou all-destroying but unconquering whale; to the last grapple with thee, from hell's heart I stab at thee; for hate's sake I spit my last breath at thee…" The harpoon was darted; the stricken whale flew forward … [and] the flying turn caught Ahab around the neck … he was shot out of the boot. … A Skyhawk that tauntingly had followed the main-truck downwards from its natural home among the stars … chanced to intercept its broad fluttering wing between the hammer and the wood … and so the bird of heaven, with archangelic shrieks, and his imperial beak thrust upwards, and his whole captive form folded in the flag of Ahab, went down with his ship, which like Satan, would not sink to hell till she had dragged a living part of heaven along with her … a sullen white surf beat against its steep sides; then all collapsed, and the great shroud of the sea rolled on as it rolled five thousand years ago. … Ishmael reports that Round and round, then, and ever contracting towards the button-like black bubble at the axis of that slowly wheeling circle … [it] did revolve. Till, gaining that vital centre, the black bubble upward burst …." (Melville, 1847/1967, pp. 468-470).

Red and white

Along with the color black of the alchemical *nigredo*, Melville plays with the other two prime colors of alchemy, with their opposition: with red and white.

In chapter 42, my favorite chapter in *Moby Dick*, "The Whiteness of the Whale," Melville plays with these two colors. I want to include examples of the author's 19th-century manner of linguistic play, his use of red and of white to impart a conscious recognition of the impact of these colors' depth, as well as their oppositional tension and attunement, their *unity and their difference*.

This colorful balance of two different entities determining the health or the well-being of the one entity can serve as a blueprint for relationships in general.

The central significance of such a colorful balance, of the right distance and closeness, the essence of any voyage to a center or a third space, or for that matter, to any healthy relationship, is meticulously circumambulated by Melville in this cogent chapter.

Clinically, Ahab is caught in a repetition compulsion, an inner scaffolding. For Ahab, this pattern is one of static opposition as well as entangled closeness. There is no dynamic relating, a dialectic, a playing contributing to a possible attunement, and—for Ahab and Moby Dick—to a possible reconciliation. I have chosen from chapter 42 but a few of these distinctly descriptive and conceptually appropriate illustrations of Ahab's too close—or too distant—relating pattern and its oppositional embedment. The two colors, red and white, act as catalysts as well as imprisoning, scaffolding vessels.

Melville views the whiteness of the whale and spotlights both the "sweet, and honorable, and sublime...[and] the [lurking] of an elusive something in the innermost idea of the hue, which strikes more of panic to the soul than that redness which affrights in blood" (Melville, 1847/1967, p. 164). The "sweet, and honorable, and sublime" of the whiteness, and the whispers of the "elusive something" remain separate for Ahab even though they could be experienced as a two in one: two oppositional forces in the one color. Reflective of the structure of his intrapsychic split, Ahab experiences in the one color, white, two estranged energies. Ahab's world does not invite a dynamic dialectic between twos.

The alchemical opposites of red and white are woven throughout *Moby Dick*, but in this chapter, Melville offers myriad illustrations of the whale's potential, yet hidden, *coniunctio* revealed in its whiteness. Were the whale setting the course, perhaps their relationship could have been an other. But for Ahab, his wound has to become the white whale's wound. This projected identification melts the two of Moby Dick and Ahab into an ossified one. There is no space for a drop of dynamic interplay between the red wound and the white whale; there is no interval for the intimate autonomy of a *coniunctio*. Ahab's color is a single, separated, alone and lonesome, solitary red. Its opposite, and therefore its antagonist, is the double threat of the whale itself plus its whiteness that hides the seductive "sublime" and the "elusive something." The first is an interpersonal projection, the latter an intrapsychic mirror.

Ahab remains too close in his identification with Moby Dick, or he is too far apart to recognize an *other*, or feel even the slightest spark of empathy. Ahab had lost a leg to Moby Dick and he remains caught in the hate and revenge of the Old Testament Law: (Exodus 21:23-25 "thou shalt give life for life,/Eye for eye ... wound for wound."). His voyage is one of retribution rather than restoration. His wound has become the whale's wound. Static and suspended on the one side in his fear of the "appalling" whiteness of the whale and at the same time, ignited by his red rage, Ahab remains stuck in this dualistic "fiery hunt" (Melville, 1847/1967, p. 170). There is no space for oppositional attunement between red and white. Ultimately, there is only one of the oppositional forces, one color, the fiery red, which consumes them. A black shroud of oceanic water from the depths opens, drenches, and devours them both. The black water then swirls them away.

Anna's and my voyage reminds me to heed the pronounced relating patterns in *Moby Dick*, to read carefully "The Whiteness of the Whale" and know the compelling nature of Ahab's red "fiery hunt." In this chapter, white and red are used primarily to obviate a more balanced relating, a relationship of conflict, movement, play and process, of attunement, a liquid relationship, and a "fiery" dialectic resolving itself into a unity of opposites, the alchemical *coniunctio*.[113]

Alchemy is grounded in matter. It is relevant to note that the relationship between red and white is grounded, in fact, in the reality of nature. Enclosed in one system, red blood cells and white blood cells are yet autonomous. These two, both red and white blood cells, are necessary for the proper functioning of the body. Red cells pick up carbon dioxide from our blood and transport oxygen, which in turn generates energy. White cells are primarily responsible for fighting foreign organisms that enter the body. Too much of either, too few of either create a dangerous and unhealthy imbalance and a high risk of ill-health. Their oppositional attunement, this balance of nature, is a determinant of health.

I would like to insert at this point a vignette, an observation, of a personal experience of the colors, red and white: their initial separation and thereafter the effect of their coming together.

Since 1999, that is, for 18 years, I had been seeing one Parkinson's specialist. To 99 percent of questions asked, his answer had been: With Parkinson's every case is different. A short time ago, he retired. At the first meeting with the new neurologist, I tell him how much better I am doing, but I note that the off times still hold me captive for hours. We talk about how this feels for me (surprise!). Then he suggests I try Amantadin. The Internet tells me it is a medication that has been prescribed for Parkinson's for years. And it is red. Most of the other medications are white. After taking Amantadin for a couple of weeks, I begin to experience a sense of harmony and balance I have not known

---

[113] Coniunctio is an alchemical operation that combines two chemicals to produce a third. Recall the "geeinte Zweinatur" of Goethe's Faust and Irigaray's "third."
"When you make the two into one, and when you make the inner like the outer and the outer like the inner, and the upper like the lower, and when you make male and female into a single one, so that the male will not be male nor the female be female, when you make eyes in place of an eye, a hand in place of a hand, a foot in place of a foot, an image in place of an image, then you will enter the Kingdom." The Gnostic Gospel of Thomas, 22. (S. Patterson & M. Meyer, Trans.). Retrieved April 27, 2018, from: http://www.gnosis.org/naghamm/gosthom.html

for years. I cannot help but wonder if the balance of the introjection of the colors red and white has not played a role in this swing into symmetry.

Is it an alchemical balance of opposites? Is there really something to this *coniunctio*, this "stone that is not a stone," this lapis of the alchemists? Or is there yet another explanation? Something to do with the plasticity of the brain? Something to do with the medication? With Anna's and my "opus"?

The whiteness of the whale

And I have not forgotten my promise to expound on the whiteness of the whale. How does white quicken? What is the relevance of white to the *Hiss of Hope*?

More important than an answer is the living with these questions, as well as with a paradox, and wondering—and watching—what the whitening reveals. Alchemically, whitening refers to the *albedo* phase of the transformative process, the experience of the consciousness gained after being burned into white ash in the preceding *nigredo* phase, the black, regressive state. A space of little ego control. Our scientist and alchemist, Newton, compares the labor of *albedo*, the alchemical silver (or white) "with the mediating action of 'Animal Spirits'…all of which work 'between' the conscious will and the physical body" (Hillman, 2009, p. 45). Does the dragonfly belong to the grouping of animal spirits? It is an insect!

White opens to reveal all the colors just as our third space unfurls when the many worlds begin to interact, when the different notes begin to resound and echoes of once-upon-a-time entities touch…and play…and dance. We know from Jung that "at the deepest level, all our 'Truths' do not emerge from our own individual experiences but from being together in the space *between*" (Jung, 1972, p. 223).[114]

---

[114] Letter to James Kirsch from Jung, "Im tiefsten Sinne traeumen wir alle nicht aus uns, sondern aus dem, was zwischen uns und dem andern liegt."

The "between" of our voyage is not a space replete with clashing differences, nor with snuggly similarities. Our voyage has taken us into the relating pattern of an intimate autonomy. A syntactical adventure, a journey beyond thought. Semantics remain onshore.

White remains on- and off-shore, it is underneath and above, visible yet invisible in its quality of presence. According to our alchemist and scientist, Isaac Newton:

> If froth be made on the surface of water thickened a little with soap, and examined closely, it will seem to be coloured with all the colours of the spectrum, but at a little distance it looks white owing to the combined effect on the eye of all the colours. (*Encyclopedia Britannica*, 1911, Vol. 19, pp. 584-585)

The dragonfly

And out of this aquatic rainbow, a dragonfly becomes visible—"a living flash of light he flew"—out of the water into the air. And "beyond the second birth of death" he flew. He flies, he darts, and he hangs in stillness.

Of course, as a libelle, or balance-fly, the two of water and of air interact, combine and change into the one, into this fascinating creature, into the dragonfly. And our white nymph, after birthing itself out of the black, first is clothed in oppositional white in order to derive from this optimal friction enough spurts of energy to fly "like a living flash of light" into a third space and fly on "thro' crofts and pastures wet with dew." For a typical nanosecond of time the incandescent wings in a flash of glowing, reddened white carry the dragonfly to a landing spot on our house where it rests before it ultimately becomes a husk—a part of the dust resting on earth's floor before the wind exhales it up to the heavens.

And thus, the tale of Ahab and Moby Dick and our voyage become woven together into an intimate autonomy. Intimate due to the dual odyssey on water, a paradigmatic symbol of the mystery of the third space when viewed in the twilight of liminality; and autonomous because after the shedding of my house-husk, and after the introjection of Anna and me, I am—like the dragonfly is a balance-fly—a *balance-person*. For the first time in my life I do not often feel threatened by imminent waves sucking me under. Nor does Parkinson's disease always grab me and torment me when high waves break. I do not feel an identification with Ahab and Moby Dick's relating pattern of imbalance and dissonance: a one without a two. Or a two without a one.

This voyage has reached a shore. Now I usually walk upon land. I *in-dwell* in my body instead of defending against the horrors of the *unknown in the water* and escaping into the air. Admittedly, I do slip on puddles once in a while, but for the most part I experience my body bending instead of Parkinson's disease freezing me into a Galatea statue.

Will this last? I do not know. Will my narcissism suck me under water again as befell Ahab and Moby Dick, and the mythological Narcissus himself? Or will I be able to remain on land more often and touch Heinz Kohut's cosmic narcissism with its qualities of "empathy, humor, creativity, an acceptance of transience, and wisdom?" (Lachmann, 2008, p. *x*)

In any case, at this point I do know that the speed of light is the only constant in the world and that my dragonfly with his flash of white light quickens me with the shafts of red movement and opens for me all the colors embedded in white, and beyond.

The narrative

This book is a scaffold of words holding me, Anna, the dragonfly, the dream entities like the pitbull, the kittens, and Melville's Ahab and his white whale together. The *"hiss* and hope" are also twos that are held together along with the third, the reflexive of no-hope, and flow into—and out of—the one. Words weave together and transport thoughts born on the inside to the outside. At the moment of *touch* between the two, the inside and the outside, a one is designed, and the third space is released. At the moment of whiteness, the alchemical *albedo*, at the moment of consciousness, the word can negate itself and is released into its truth. "With the speed of light it flies"—and like the color white, whose light is capable of exciting the sensation of vision, a word is "released into its truth" and is then seen. And now comes relationship—or not.

I have translated the following story from a book for children "who like to draw." The inspiration comes from Faust, who was willing to regress into a space of nothingness and discovers that it is not empty. Rather, through reduced ego control, Faust is to experience everything (*alles*). In this German drama, *alles* is seen in Faust's experience of the relating pattern of an intimate autonomy in the love between the mythological couple, Paris and Helen. Faust's regression offers him the opportunity to view things in a new light, in a new color.

> *"Let's go for it! I want to get at the bottom of all this.*
> *In your nothingness, I hope to discover everything!"*
> (Goethe, 1806/1992)[115]

In this book, the story of white offers the reader the opportunity to view this color through new eyes.

The True Story of All Colors

In the Beginning was White. When you see that everything is open, bright and clean, then it is White. The first color to appear after white is Red. Red proclaims in a loud voice: "I am here now. Pay attention to me! Is there someone else here other than me?" White replied; "Yes, I am here." "Ach," said Red. "I hadn't noticed you!" This is due to the fact that White is so very modest. Without admitting it, Red knows that White is there. He is aware that he gains a certain glow, when White is present. All the colors do. It

---

[115] "Nur immerzu. Wir wollen es ergruenden./ In deinem Nichts, hoffe ich das All zu finden!" (Faust, lines 6255, 6256)

wasn't long before the other colors appear. Each color declares its prime importance and each color insists that it be presented as the most vital. It isn't long before a fierce fight ensues. The longer the battle rages, the darker everything becomes. Soon there is only Black. Even Blue with her deep wisdom does not know what to do next. At that moment Blue feels desperate and calls out from the darkness: "Help! Can someone help us? We have all disappeared into the Blackness." Suddenly, a strange sound is heard. A sort of liquid "bloop." It sounded like a scoop of whipped cream being tossed onto a plate. "You have called me, and I have come," affirmed White. Exhausted, the other colors all crawl out of the Blackness. "Stop!" White called out. "You must leave each other's space. Otherwise, you will all once again disappear into Darkness." "The other colors should just disappear," shouted Red. "I was here before they were!" "No!" declared White. "Each color is equally important. Each color deserves its own space. Each color must be autonomously respected at the same time that each of you are intimately close. We are going to have a Color Wheel. The structure of this Wheel will contain each of you separately, but at the same time, it will demand that each respect the other's space." Simultaneously the Color Wheel prevents entanglement. "You are not too close, nor too separate. None of you will fall into Blackness." And with these words, and with the immediate advent of the Color Wheel, White disappears once again. But its light remains. (Heller, 1994)

****

And with the geometrical form, the color wheel, a new sketch of the relating pattern of an intimate autonomy is introduced. And the dance begins.

The once-upon-a-time nymph that has transmuted into a mercurial dragonfly is my partner at the moment. Its hermetic wings carry my words, my thoughts, from the inside to the outside, from me to you, and from "us" to the world. And out of the world. Currently, I am in the process of "emergence…searching for a safe place away from the water…the skin begins to split…the adult pushes up and out of the

239

skin…sometimes falling back into the water…if flight is attempted too soon, there can be existential damage" (Mitchell & Lasswell, 2005, pp. 55-85). The heart of the dragonfly is my spirit, its self-unfolding pattern, my pulsating core. The eyes of the dragonfly are my intuition: its body, my illness, and my "higher health."

Emergence into the adult phase

The dance

Emergence into the adult phase feels like a centripetal core force pulling everything together while it simultaneously plays with a protective scaffold that centrifugally sustains like skin. It feels like a rhythmic pull and release dynamic. Like riding the waves of an ocean. Like feeling in intimate contact with the wave and then suddenly being swept into an autonomy where there is nothing but air. After this interlude of little motion, another wave engulfs me. It throws me up. Just when I become used to the surge of water, I am tossed into oceans of still energy. Back and forth and forth and back. We play. The water and me. And the air.

If I were to imagine a dialectical dance between the energies of intimacy and autonomy, it would be a dance that takes place in one and in all organisms. If I were to attempt to construct a structural relating pattern that reflects a general energetic interaction between opposites or between twos—like the two: intimacy and autonomy—it would be a choreographed configuration resembling rhythms and cadences endemic to a birth process. The wrenching physical pain, the occasional existential fear, the physical as well as the psychological vulnerability demanded are instances of motion and form sketching the inception of life's dance. Between the biologically initiated dance patterns are the generated aggressive, self-assertive moments of ego activity: the physical pushing.

These are moments unraveled from the more general process of a two emerging out of a one; that is, the baby being birthed into a two, out of feeling like a one with the mother while in the womb. The concluding formation of the dance of intimate autonomy is the emergence of a two from one. And a one from two. A two that quickly attaches again and becomes the two as one it once was. Life's dance is a flow from intimacy to autonomy, back and forth and forth and back. There are the clashing, connecting moments—the paradoxical intimate autonomy—without which there would be no dance. With a nod of my head and a grin on my face, I assume the role of choreographer.

***

The following interlude contains the anthropomorphism of our two words: *intimate autonomy*. They are going to be configured as two partners in a dance. The choreography presents them as twos, or opposites in relationship. Unable to be in any kind of relationship, they fight or flight or freeze in order to avoid a dialogue. Until, quite by chance, they experience a moment of being a one. And they unfold into an intimate autonomy, a relating pattern of paradox, of flow, a configuration of love and of truth.

"…come dance with me…"

Intimacy bows and makes the first advance. *Autonomy* quickly retreats. She pursues him. He reacts by trying to disappear. In her need for more closeness, she relentlessly continues her attack. *Autonomy* eventually capitulates. For a second. And then he turns the tables and avows to frighten her away. In a startlingly fast turnabout, he becomes the pursuer. The power shifts into its opposite. What was previously the perpetrator becomes the victim. *Intimacy* fears *Autonomy*. It is not long before *Autonomy* becomes complacently assured of dominating the dance. She yields. But it is a farce. This dance is a travesty of a relation-ship, she realizes. *Intimacy* turns and, bursting with anger, she challenges him to stop moving, to meet her face to face, and to allow an encounter, even a confrontation. At least it would be a relationship of sorts. The unexpected startles him to fall back. Quickly he catches himself and, with a nod to the mystery of "curiosity," *Autonomy* simply stops. Movement ceases in the center; energy seems to be put on hold. A paradox: an *intimate autonomy*?

The dance, however, continues. But there is no visible movement. There is no discernible motion. But there *is* an amalgamation, a slight coalescence, a whisper of vertical and horizontal lines crossing. And at the exact point of this crossing, the two become a one. It is a kairos moment, a syzygy, the key to a whole new world: the potential space of a paradox, an equipoise. A flash…and then the dance of Twos (or more) commences once again. And again. And again …The moments of the Oneness can incarnate in a cascading swirl of a waltz, a moment of remaining *autonomous* while simultaneously sinking into an animating *intimacy*. At this moment, the center of the dance spaces, oneness becomes for our two—*intimacy* and *autonomy*—the place of paradox, yet also of relationship. The dance continues diffused with a new kind of energy.

A paradox most often is assumed to signal a cessation of energy between opposites. In the case of our *intimately autonomous* relating pattern, it can herald instead a possible surge of consciousness, of a new space, of daring to be together. Perhaps even to love. Or to hope.

This dance never ceases.

***

In every dance set, both intimacy and autonomy know that each gives into—and unto—the other. Each knows that in this moment of opening and yielding, the exposure and the vulnerability generate oppositional dynamism, that just the right distance and just the right closeness have to be sensed. At this moment, a maturity is bestowed, and both energies weep drops of joy. A kind of ectoplasmic viscous substance is discovered on each tear. There are visible traces of ectoplasm to be found in particular regions of the ocean.

My dance into an intimate autonomy:
A reflection of the dragonfly

"The final molt into the adult stage....If the larva successfully
finds a safe place away from the water, its legs stiffen and lock
to the surface it is resting upon. Then emergence begins..."
(Mitchell & Lasswell, 2005, pp. 67, 71).

Early one morning Anna and I leave the upstairs bedroom area and go
downstairs to the kitchen. Everything happens so fast: Anna slips and
begins to fall head first down the stairs. I am in front of her. A mirror of
the dragonfly's emergence into its adult phase, my *"legs stiffen and lock
to the surface."* Feeling totally calm and *knowing* in this present moment
of the secure attachment of my legs to the stairs, of the strength of my
body, and of the centripetal core force, I intercept and detain Anna's
fall, which otherwise could have propelled her head first down the rest
of the long, winding staircase.

I note the energies between Anna and me. I could revel in the
fugitive autonomy and momentarily ignore any repetitive compulsive
structural nonintimacy with her and with Parkinson's disease. Instead,
the clean clarity of being with Anna and equally with myself feels just
right. Have the syntactical entities of the structure, the pattern and the
networking of the relating pattern of an intimate autonomy, spun a
web of glass simulating themselves again and again until sundry other
relationships become a firm one and two, a dance of paradoxical
conflict, collision, and incongruity, yet often also resounding reflections
of the joy of parity heard like a symphony of strings played on
instruments of glass? And ubiquitously inexorable?

The second noteworthy change and potential hint of my own
emergence into the adult phase of the voyage is likewise physical. And
correspondingly mirroring the dragonfly once again, it is a body
concern.

A strikingly common symptom of Parkinson's disease is constipation. For years since the onset of Parkinson's disease, my body has

held on tightly and has required the help of prunes and Metamusil to let loose after three or four days. A shift to the internal releasing, which allows the more normal daily stool, is sudden, and for me this loosening of an inner bowel function is encouraging. I have imagined that the off-and-on jerky movement disorder phases of Parkinson's that have obstinately persisted in turning me into a statue, and then suddenly releasing me, would now begin to relinquish their dualistic boomerang grip. When constipation loosens and yields its rigid immobility, spaces are opened, core areas become available to *chi* energy. With the guidance and mercurial flexibility of this central force, a gradual transmutation of Parkinson's off-versus-on opposition is effected.

The embedded desperate pattern of dualism, this primally wrought pattern of *relationlessness,* or a too-close structural pattern, the stuck repetition compulsion of Parkinson's' on/off separateness, as well as any either/or begins to morph into a dynamic intimate autonomy. A sense of a relaxing into a kind of chaos rather than remaining imprisoned in my more recurrent dualistic split. Chaos is open; chaos portends potential creativity. The relationship between my brain and my body, the structural trajectories of Parkinson's, can now sense another possible form of communication and thus lure and stimulate the plasticity of the brain to interiorize and engage itself in a process of metamorphosis.

Perhaps Parkinson's loud, dissonant screams can be reduced to the euphonic murmur of a prayer. The viaduct of this metamorphosis would then have been something as innately basic to me and to the dragonfly as our common excrement and our intimate yet autonomous trans-formations of mirrored launchings into the adult phase.

Perhaps the spirit of the dragonfly has orchestrated my emergence and, specifically, this onset. For the dragonfly, the physical control over his feces is unique. A core feature of its ripening into the adult phase includes being able to sense how to use the small pellets formed from fecal matter: It can either eject them when it wants to skim over water as fast as possible, or it can contain the pellets when a mosquito flies around and it wants to be still and focused. With the hunter's dance of concentrated stillness, it can then catch its prey.

Mirroring the dragonfly's maturation, I observe these first two reflective hints of my own emergence: the firm strength in my legs and body, and the seemingly opposite inner loosening of the bowel tract. Both are now held together by a new core, a newly constituted centripetal center, a source of passionate focus the dragonfly seemingly never has had to sacrifice. It has simply always had this wellspring, this insect-instinctual primal vital center, a fiery force that can quicken and forge life's patterns. In addition, such a center opens to a place where the dragonfly can gather stillness. From the same source the dragonfly seems to gather sparks to take off into the air like a flash of lightning (or like Superman!).

Also indicative of a dragonfly's instinctual guidance, a physical expulsion quite foreign from my usual head—or morally based behavior—is that words seem to fly out of my mouth, words that normally would be consciously—and most likely unconsciously—censored. One example stands out: As usual, Anna is driving, as usual I am putting my feet on imaginary brakes when we pull up to a four-way stop. Waiting there is one other car. When this car does not immediately begin to move, I hear myself say aggressively: "*Fahr, du Bloede!*" (Drive, you stupid nut!). Anna is still laughing about that. But the mirth is mixed with a recognition of the emergence of a part of me hitherto denied and split off. Looking back at the feeling accompanying these words, I recognize the surprising presence of the pitbull.

Yet an additional hint of portending ripening into my adult phase has been a major inner restructuring. I have grown up with such koans as "it rains louder at night" or "at night one can hear one hand clapping." Without any real comprehension, I know that perception during the night differs from daytime consciousness. Despite these Zen sparks of wisdom, I am not prepared for the thoroughly alien and violent takeover of Parkinson's disease and its vicious nightly visitations. As noted before, whereas my nights had been spaces of rest and of revivification, with the invasive advent of Parkinson's, they become spaces of submission, helplessness, and endurance. Whereas I had been able to glide from a daylight disbursement of energy into a nightly reimbursement, post-Parkinson's condemns me not only to an empty energetic balance sheet, but it doles out short sleep spaces, the most opulent being 90 minutes. Almost on the exact end of the half hour, Parkinson's suddenly interrupts my sleep with various wake-up calls. One I term "the jackhammer" because my body suddenly begins to shake with such intense rhythmic force that it feels like street cement is cracked open and broken through again and again. Or Parkinson's initiates the sudden spasmodic seizures of restless leg syndrome. Or the long immobility of my right leg or shoulder causes them both to suddenly scream with the shock of burning pain.

Once again, the movement disorder of Parkinson's disease reveals oppositional structures, stubborn syntactical noncommunication. The early morning ritualistic gymnastics necessary to glide out of the statuesque nightly immobility has increased in time involvement as well as energy expenditure. I used to be able to become free after about 30 minutes. Now I need at least 90 minutes.

I used to always love early morning jogging.

In the present stage of my emergence, my nights are still not easy, but comparatively I have fewer and less violent wake-up calls, I can often sleep two hours now. I have discovered T. S. Eliot's "dance" at the "still point": It is a dance of happiness when quickened by the Zen-splash of a cool sun-drenched waterfall in the midst of nightly wanderings in the wilderness. A dream drenched by the subjective gyrations of the water drops falling on me from the sea or splashing from a waterfall on to land, I am in a space of stillness. But in this still space I do not dance. I am a danced-object—perhaps like the dragonfly. And being the object instead of the subject (the determining ego) feels ironically perhaps like freedom. Like not being transformed into a marble statue. Like not being Galatea.

From a dream space of relative egolessness, there have been additional hints of emergence: I've noticed that the syntax of my dreams has changed. They are no longer filled with sequences of the movement of persons breaking into my house, coming through the walls of my apartment. No longer am I desperately running—and sometimes flying—away from abusive, violent men chasing me. Instead, I remember vividly being with a black-and-white striped kitten throughout a long dream, a kitten that I hold close to my breast. I am determined to protect it from all possible harm. And at this point, the dream unfolds to let in feelings, to let in semantics: For this striped kitten I feel a new kind of involuntary love, a connection that envelops me in a feeling of security and safety even though, paradoxically, it is the kitten I know to protect and to keep from harm. Is this the hint of a life I have yet to feel: the intimacy and attachment for the infant on the weighing scale? For Winnicot's "true me"? For yet one more *with* I am to fathom?

In other dreams, I am busy building a new house or renovating an apartment. In one dream, there is a hand slowly passing in front of my eyes. It is looking at me through its own eyes! Later, I recall Rilke's "Archaic Torso of Apollo" and his poetic lines:

> *"... Yet*
> *his torso, like a lamp, still glows*
> *with his gaze which, although turned down low,*
> *lingers and shines...*
> *like starlight: for there's not one spot*
> *that doesn't see you. You must change your life...."* [116]

The hand is open and is holding a fully blooming red rose. In the dream, I recall once again the words of Winnicott: "as an adult you will bloom like a rose, or unripen into a bud."

In the dream, I feel a quality of presence, a gaze to low gleams, a sense of the two stripes of the kitten conversing with each other and often panting common meows of hope. A sense of a future.

Nights float past. Like the dragonfly, I feel like I am "pushing up and out of my old skin...it is prone to damage if it (the dragonfly) flies before drying" (Mitchell & Lasswell, 2005, p. 71). The dragonfly has to

---

[116] The relevant portion of "The Archaic Torso of Apollo" (my translation and the German version) is located in Appendix A-10.

247

wait until the wings are full of blood and oxygen, until its wings can carry it. I wait.

Then suddenly, I am shoved into a potential frighteningly fugitive onset of autonomy by those with whom I am most intimately involved.

A fugitive autonomy

On one sunny Friday afternoon, Anna begins to complain of acute stomach pains. She begins to look pale; the pains increase. Despite her protests, my husband and I call an ambulance and she is taken to the hospital. And she is admitted. The diagnosis is pancreatitis and gallbladder stones. The complete area, including the liver, is infected.

For three days, Anna hovers between life and death.

During these days and nights, I sense a faint flutter of dragonfly wings. As if they do not know what to do. A space of chaos. No net. The old repetition compulsion of the Snow Queen split: She does not have to feel anything? She is in control. Or this new space of unknown trajectories, of wings carrying me forth—I know not where. And Rilke's words in his *First Elegy*: "every angel is terrifying."

With Anna in the hospital, my husband has sole care of me. After a night of my constant demands on his time and on his physical strength, he tells me that he feels that he is sacrificing his own health. He does not want to care for me anymore. I feel the familiar old repetitive patterns of icy sharp claws of abandonment. They begin to claw away at me. My old protective scaffold has been ripped off of me instead of my shedding it. I am exposed, naked, and terrified. Helpless.

Looking back later on this stage of the morphology, I suddenly grasp that this kind of regression, which opens potential meta-morphoses, contains a centrifugal psychic force that, like a virus, infects others. Not only have I, myself, been tossed about in the waves of our anaclitic therapy, but those intimately involved are likewise on/in and under the water of this voyage. And Anna and my husband have also both been thrown up and down by the waves and are often unwillingly swept away by the strong currents of the undertow.

With rest, antibiotics, and emotional support from us, from friends, and relatives in Germany, and special support from one child, 8 years old, for whom Anna has been a baby whisperer, after 14 days of hospital care, Anna's health returns.

My husband, on the other hand, has emerged from this fear of losing himself in the process of giving to me with experiences of—perhaps one could use the word *yogic* to define this—healthy although difficult stretching he has experienced. Following his initial desperation and withdrawal from the caregiver position, he begins to attend yoga classes four or five times a week and has assumed a new position. There seems to be an available central wellspring in him that he begins to tap. Or perhaps the opposites of stretching and relaxing into this same stretch have opened a new trajectory, a new potential pattern of communication between previous oppositional forces. In any case, in our voyage there is another compelling energy at work now. At the present, he radiates a new calmness and a centripetally compelling glow that draws one to him rather than the previous, more protective energy that portends flares of impending anger and often holds others at bay.

Perhaps as a byproduct of my original experience of violent abandonment, and due to Anna and my anaclitic therapy as well as her and my husband's reorganizations, Parkinson's likewise has undergone structural changes. The disease's ons and offs opposition, Parkinson's dualistic structural frame, has softened, and a kind of inner intermittent dialogue seems to have begun. Wrenched from its repetition compulsive nature of rendering me either immobile or not, Parkinson's internal dialogue reflects outward and—like a mirror catching the sun—I am *burned* into a different way of moving. My kinetic energy is different: I flow instead of jerk. I am no longer embedded in a movement-disorder split where I am catapulted from one opposite to the other. There is now a gentler, more orderly, flow underlying my walking and my physical movements in general. The former oppositional dualism has opened to allow different rhythms, varied paths, and new physical avenues for me to explore.

249

An additional hint of emergence is the sudden and painful cut of the glass threads of defensive patterns, the tenuous and fugitive containment of the split, and of dualistic relating. There is a new distance between Anna and me, and between my husband and me. And between me and not-me, there is a foreign yet underpinning density. A closeness that is not too close, not entangled. Perhaps it is a new inner (and outer) movement. Not yet familiar. At times frightening. For both Anna and my husband, I feel gratitude and a fresh kind of love for both. Not primarily because of their love and their care for me as much as an appreciation for their ability to be loved.

My thoughts wander through misty nets while gathering light and clarity.

There are three stages in the life of the dragonfly: the egg, the larva or nymph stage, and the adult stage. In the water, the egg stage can last longer than 4 years; as a nymph the dragonfly molts up to 17 times before emerging as an adult. In most species of dragonflies, the larval stage lasts longer than the adult stage; it is certainly much longer than most larva stages of other insects...it takes a median of 14.2 days for a male dragonfly to reach sexual maturity once it has emerged to the adult stage. The dragonflies that have survived this period can live for 11 days longer, or a total of 25 days. Maximum life spans are believed to be a little less than 40 days. The dragonfly's last transmutation into an adult is perhaps the most difficult and the most meaningful. (Mitchell & Lasswell, 2005, p. 67-98)

Exemplifying the intimate yet autonomous relating patterns, adult dragonflies do not tolerate captivity of any kind. Their relationships with each other are not of significant duration. They are intimately attached to each other when mating, but soon thereafter they part. The structure of an intimate autonomy is an interpersonal as well as an intrapsychic syntax threading itself throughout the life of the dragonfly. The more autonomous life of the adult seems to depend on the extended time of the more intimate preparation. Even the onset of adult life can be viewed as a monklike meditative withdrawal, an intimate being with itself, before any mature autonomy can be experienced. If the dragonfly flies too soon, before his wings are filled with blood and with oxygen, and have dried, it is fatal. A fairly exact balancing act between intimacy and autonomy, between doing and being, is one of dragonfly's unique innate propensities toward reaching the adult stage.

Once seen and experienced, the incandescent glow of the dragonfly remains, however, even though the dragonfly itself soon dies after the emergence into the adult phase. The dragonfly's relatively long voyage in the larval stage and its short life as an adult mirror truths about a journey being more significant than the goal. The dragonfly's fiery passionate spirit and the luminescent and intricate singular beauty of its wings ensure a lasting impression of an ephemeral being.

The word

My task as an energy is likewise to maintain the structural relating pattern of an intimate autonomy in my relationship to the word and to my writing. While writing, I have noted that the flow begins when I open an intimate door to the inside of the word, and try to know its autonomy, its *Urwort* (primal word). Indeed, I do not open this door. I wait...and wait...and wait. Sometimes, again I become the object; the door itself opens, and I dare to enter. A simultaneous rush of wind through time and the gasp of my breath signal at least a second's experience of hearing the vibrations of the *Urwort* reverberating through the centuries. I recognize a moment's emergence into the adult stage: My ego does not have to maintain control.

And as for Parkinson's, I feel less compelled to preside over this disease, and ironically perhaps I feel more able to be flashed through life like the dragonfly yet sometimes even to emulate its stillness; even a deathlike stillness is becoming possible. And I ponder once again T. S. Eliot's words in "Burnt Norton":

> ...except for the still point
> there is no dance.
> And there is only the dance.

And I watch myself and the wind. And the sun. As an adult, am I now able to "stand naked in the wind"? And can I allow myself now to "melt into the sun" (Gibran, 1932)?

Time has passed. Anna has returned to Germany. There is no return date set. Do I still need her, or can I just enjoy her without the searing and frightening feeling of abandonment, or its precipitating too-closeness? Indeed, I want to just enjoy the stillness and the dance of an intimate autonomy shared with her.

The hiss of hope (I)

I think my wings have dried; my words have become at least partially filled with blood and with oxygen. But I can hear strange, often foreign, words breathing. Some of them are not my words. Nor are they the wings of the dragonfly. They seem to fly upon the paper of their own free will. Or I catch myself uttering words I would consciously reject. Jungian *shadow* words. Sometimes like "a flash of light," words sparkle, an epiphanic thought emerges. Then it just disappears. And no matter how intensely I try to think, remembering is impossible. It feels as if the words are playing…or they are dancing …with me, with the dragonfly, with themselves. They are there and they are not there.

But where do they come from, what is their space of origin?

Perhaps there is no space of origin. Instead, as "a living flash of light," energy moves. A thought is born and is exteriorized along the trajectories of language. And then it settles in stillness on the paper and crystallizes into a word. Its movement is not a movement disorder, Parkinson's disease's epithet. Instead, words descend with the indemnity of musical notes ordering themselves onto the lines of compositional scores, like rhythmic water drops either falling from the wings of a dragonfly or splashing off from playful oceanic waves. There is often a tinge of red in these drops, or veins of black. I hear dissonant atonal sounds when the white whale warns of the embedded *hiss* in hope, of the inevitable descent of the sudden searing tears of *hiss*, were I to imprison myself in future hope and lose no-hope. From the depths, the whale warns me of the seduction of semantics; he implores me to sustain the autonomy of the structural syntax of relating between hope and no-hope—these two—intimately attached. And to listen for the *hiss*.

There is a sudden flash of light, and I notice the two touch, and there is a moment of one when a new, an untried, dance begins. An unfamiliar configuration, a new word is unveiled. I taste no *hiss*; I feel no hope. But I hear a whisper: the breath of an untried word.

Epilogue

Dragonfly eyes

Contemporary interest in the eyes of the dragonfly has yielded compelling results. The dragonfly's relating pattern with light, with color, and with movement, its sense of concentrated discernment and navigational acuity when pursuing prey astonishes entomologists. Recent research reveals the possibility of calculating algorithmic operations based on dragonfly's vision that can help the eyesight of people who can see nothing. This same system is expected to find applications in automated technologies that rely on artificial sight, such as robots and driverless cars.

Dragonflies are true visionaries. Their eyes are the keenest in the insect world. Indeed, perhaps also in the human world. Dragonflies have visual senses that would be considered superpowers by any human standards. They seem to be able to "see" even "beyond," for a dragonfly knows exactly when to cease to feed several days before it leaves the water and emerges out of its larva. (Bagheri, Wiederman, Cazzolato, Grainger, & O'Carroll, 2015, n.p.)[117]

---

[117] In this Journal of the Royal Society Interface, scientists show how a computer program can mirror the eyesight of a dragonfly. The discovery can be integrated into bionic eyes, which use a retinal implant connected to a video camera to convert images into electrical impulses that carry signals back to the brain. Simulating a dragonfly's 360-degree field of vision and tracking ability could help visually impaired people sense when someone unexpectedly walks into their path, for example. "The dragonfly catches prey at speeds up to 60 kilometers/37 miles/per hour, capturing them with a success rate of 97%...." In California,

My eyes

I have just had two cataract operations, first my left eye and then, two weeks later, my right eye. Both Anna and my husband are with me for the two operations. After a five-month hiatus at home in Germany, Anna has returned to Edmonton and plans to be here for five weeks.

According to the dictionary, *cataract* not only refers to an impairment of vision but also alludes to a waterfall, a sudden rush of water, a cascade of white water. The prevalent understanding of a cataract, however, is a clouding of the lens inside the eye that leads to

---

for example, one company, Second Sight Medical Products Inc., has approval to market its retinal prosthesis in the U.S. to treat a specific type of blindness. A video camera embedded in a pair of eyeglasses can gather visual input in the form of light and transmit it to the implant as an electrical signal.

I have gleaned from various contemporary articles and books (The Dazzle of Dragonflies) some relevant and interesting facts about dragonflies:

The eyes of a dragonfly make me feel weird when I look at them. The pseudopupils, the dark points in the eyes, move as the head turns, and I feel as if I am being observed no matter where I go. These individual single eyes, the ommatidium, are each supplied with a nerve connection and each sees. Yet all function together as a unit. A composite image is formed. With these unique attributes, the dragonfly has unusual vision.

Each of these compound eyes of the dragonfly is composed of several thousand elements known as facets (or ommatidia) that contain certain light-sensitive proteins, thereby functioning as the visual sensing element in the compound eye. Their eyes are the largest of any insect, each eye containing up to 30,000 facets. Each facet creates its own image, and the dragonfly brain has eight pairs of descending visual neurons to compile those thousands of images into one picture. Dragonflies can detect the plane of polarization of light, which humans cannot do without the aid of sunglasses.

Another visual advantage of the multifaceted eye of the dragonfly is its acute sensitivity to movement. They manage to snatch their targets in midair more than 95 percent of the time. Recent research has pinpointed key features of the dragonfly's brain, eyes, and wings that allow it to hunt so unerringly. One hypothesis is that the nervous system of the dragonfly displays an almost human capacity for selective attention and is able to focus on a single prey as it flies. Perhaps the way a guest at a party can attend to a friend's words while ignoring background chatter.

Other researchers—including Robert M. Olberg of Union College, Proceedings of the National Academy of Sciences—have identified a kind of master circuit of 16 neurons that connect the dragonfly's brain to its flight motor center in the thorax. With the aid of that neuronal package, the dragonfly can track a moving target, calculate a trajectory to intercept that target and, subtly adjust its path as needed.

Human eyes have three opsins—which sense light—giving us a color range of red, green, and blue (one for each opsin). Dragonfly eyes can have four or five. They can perceive the normal color spectrum along with the UVI light and the plane of light polarization.

a decrease in vision. The word *cataract* is derived from the Latin *cataracta*, meaning "waterfall" and from the ancient Greek *katarrhaktes*, "down-rushing." As rapidly running water turns white, so the term may have been used metaphorically to describe the similar appearance of mature ocular opacities. Early Persian physicians called the term *nazul-i-ah*, or "descent of the water," believing such blindness to be caused by an outpouring of corrupt humor, or "bile," into the eye.[118] This belief continued to be widespread until far into the 19th century, when medical research began to question such theories. Now bile is more often used to mean anger or irritability, depression, or even soap that removes various kinds of tough stains.

Before the first operation begins, the surgeon tells me to watch the light. I know that light enters the eye through a lens to create an upside-down image that the brain turns right-side up. While I ponder this relating pattern between the eye and the brain, the surgeon touches my head and holds it for a few seconds. Parkinson's feels contained and does not try a Hermeslike dragonfly sudden twist to fly out of the situation. The doctor tells me afterward that he is amazed how still I am when he touches me. This is the first eye, the left one. The right eye is to follow in two weeks.

The light during the first operation lures me into an intense experience of unity. Again, like Ahab's relating pattern of identification with the whale! As in Ahab's life, so in his death. He and the white whale are as if tethered together by Ahab's harpoon, and then, as a welded one, they disappear and seem to dissolve in the swirling black oceanic waters.

The oneness I know, too. But then it often jerks suddenly into its opposite: the vertical split. Me into a separated two.

---

[118] The four distinct bodily fluids in a person—known as humors—are in balance if the person is healthy. And in Western culture the historical concept of balance is a widespread goal to reach. In the past it was believed that all diseases and disabilities resulted from an excess or deficit of one of these four humors. The four humors are black bile—black (earth); yellow bile—yellow (fire); phlegm—purple (water); and blood—red (air). From Hippocrates onward, Greek, Roman, and Persian physicians adopted this theory, and it became the most commonly held view among European physicians until the advent of modern medical research in the 19th century.

In this moment of being an object operated upon, I split and escape the actual physicality, the somatic pain. I leave my body. And I become one with the light. I feel like Luke Skywalker in *Star Wars*, flying around space guided by the Force. I am the Force and I am the Light. I fly and fly…and then, suddenly, it is all over. And I walk out to where Anna and my husband are waiting, as if nothing has happened.

From the onset of the second operation two weeks later, I sense that this encounter is going to be different. Objectively, the second operation unfolds mirroring the first. But subjectively, I seem to be in a different world. Following the surgeon's instructions once again to attend to the light, I do so. The surgeon is the same. His words and his hand on my head are identical to the time before. Fugitive thoughts about upside-down gingerbread or about the intimately autonomous relating pattern between the eye and the brain are also there.

The light is the same and not the same. I am the same and not the same. The Force has abandoned me. (Or I have abandoned the Force.) The light begins to assume a reddish hue at the same moment that I feel the surgeon penetrating my eye with a sharp instrument. I *feel* the cutting into my eye; I *feel* "blood" running down my cheek—a sudden rush of liquid, perhaps a "cascade of white *and red* water." I experience time, the approximate 20 minutes necessary for the removal of the old and the planting of the new lens. And then it's finally over. I feel irritable.

I am on earth. I feel more connected to matter, to my body, safer perhaps, more contained in a world net. More ability to withstand "reality"? And the light…I see differently. It feels as if my one eye and the second eye are *seeing* together for the first time. And yet more. I see from behind my eyes. And the light…the light is different. It feels like a recollection of scattered units or sparks of light into an ordered, centered unity.

I've heard of an alchemical ingredient called *caelum*, a pale blue liquid, a mixture of various ingredients from the earth and from the heavens, a "universal form, containing in itself all forms, distinct from one another, but proceeding from one single universal form…a dew of the sea," that is associated with "divine grace that drips from the moon." I see as through a "pureness floating to the top, transparent, shining, and of the color of purest air" (Edinger, 1995, pp. 111, 287, 291). In *Endymion*, Keats describes it as

> *"An endless fountain of immortal drink,*
> *Pouring unto us from heaven's brink…"*

Each of these tiny facets of the dragonfly eye faces a different direction and each produces a tiny image. The insect brain puts all of these tiny images together to form a picture….

It has taken me many years to be able to not only see the stars in the heavens but also to note and be able to look at the bile on earth. It has taken me years to be able to wander in the red and the black of the wilderness on earth and to recognize that I can survive. It has taken me years to be able to see and to relate to the red anger of the pitbull without immediately having to split off and head for the soft muted light and safety of the gentle, adapted kitten. It has taken years of enduring the pain of being a prisoner of the vertical split's structural boomerang, being tossed back and forth and forth and back from one opposite to another. Somehow, somewhere, my brain has reorganized itself, and with the new lens of the second operation, the cataract cascades in an explosion of white fury from my eye, and at the same time, playing with the unfamiliar light, I can be intimate with the blood red color when I sense the freed liquid stream down my cheek.

Repetition compulsion

The heavy scaffolding of the repetition compulsive structural pattern of protective splitting seems to be at least partially sacrificed. It's not anymore a matter of being Luke Skywalker in a vertical split and feeling nothing; nor the other possibility of being "on earth" and contending with the red fury of the pitbull. Perhaps now I can—like the dragonfly—put these different images together and envision dancing with any twos— or more—on the firm yet paradoxically liquid foundation of one picture.

Before the washing or cleansing of the second cataract operation, the fear of the pain endemic to closeness, to intimacy, has prohibited seeing a two in one as anything other than an annihilating relating pattern. I can glimpse an intimate autonomy's paradoxical pattern of a simultaneous closeness and distance, the possibility of a dance with both Luke and with the pitbull, but it remains an abstract notion. Fear concedes true visibility only to the one eye. The singularity of this frozen separation has been the only relating pattern I have been able to tolerate. The protective landscape has been where water becomes crystal, the sun becomes ice, the moon becomes silver, and time stands still. In this split terrain, Parkinson's has lived and flourished, while its patterned movement disorder renders me immobile and closes true visibility.

More than 80 percent of the dragonfly brain is devoted to analyzing visual information. Eighty percent! Wow! I begin to analyze this visual information, the colors, the new living *on earth*, the newly discovered pattern of two eyes relating to each other, while simultaneously envisioning one image. Then I remember the dragonfly and its insect brain. This brain, that is the size of a grain of rice, does not actually analyze, it does not think. It allows the images to be arranged (or to arrange themselves?), like the pixels of a computer or a television shape and form a picture. Do electric impulses whisper algorithms to those listening dots?

I try to consciously relax my controlling ego. I also set aside my love of thought and of analysis. Almost immediately, I sense a withdrawal of my surroundings. I hear noise as through a filter. My lungs breathe. And I become my breath. My hitherto occupied space empties. I have never felt able to tolerate the energy, the dynamic, the intensity of an unscaffolded space, of a space of naked nothingness. Now, for the first time in my life I do not experience the nothingness filling with debilitating anxiety. Nor do I know my ego to panic and desperately fill the vacuum with me and nothing but me. Nor do I become immobile at the sight of red.

Looking through eyes facing myriad directions simultaneously, *knowing* that the images *seen* are held together by a point in a center, processing with the most primitive of instinctual insect thinking, having emerged from the darkness of an egg through its crack to light, to water, and to life, the dragonfly recognizes the fomenting influence of dark and light on each other. It actually comes into contact with the dialectic dance of opposites. The dragonfly sees that darkness and light relate to each other like fluid oppositional forces. It experiences their dynamic connection and sees that each one of the two undergoes a basic rearrangement. The darkness can weaken the light in its working power. Conversely, the light can limit the energy of the darkness. In both cases, something new is created: untried hues, modulated tones, result.[119]

An unfamiliar relating pattern has cascaded down into the chasm of the vertical split. My reality has been realigned: There are at least two now. They influence each other's quality of presence by the mutual infusion of a new sensation, an unaccustomed awareness.

Parkinson's disease

Parkinson's is a chronic movement disorder, which means that the relationship between it and me usually becomes gradually more and more unbalanced. "Chronic" suggests that it is my fate to have Parkinson's assume an ever-increasing dominating role over me. Parkinson's disease has forced me to see "bile" in my body as well as darkness on earth. Subjectively, I am now able to recognize my anchoring anger at Parkinson's violent and intrusive invasion. Its gradual yet indefatigably impolite and autocratic takeover has changed my life.

With the viciously invasive cutting through of my life's structural patterns, the slicing of my ego into tiny pieces, the callous curtailment of my plans and hopes, with the *hiss* of Eve's snake and the ancient wisdom of my dragonfly, Parkinson's disease has managed to generate and to quicken a silvery slithering dialectic between previously frozen opposites. And with the cascade of white and red water rushing down my cheek, I am swept into a life hitherto unknown.

Since the beginning of anaclitic therapy and the gradual unfolding of the relating pattern with Anna, Parkinson's and my relating pattern have assumed a different configuration, a more fuguelike equality perhaps. My

---

[119] See Goethe's Farbenlehre.

movements have become less disorderly. My movements have become less entangled; my mobility, my ability to move, has increased. Parkinson's seems deliberately to have become less cruel and violent.

This disease has adjusted the protective scaffolding of the clinical split, the separation whose defensive function has protected me all my life, while simultaneously generating an anxiety often paralyzing in its egregious, ubiquitous attacks. Furthermore, Parkinson's has set free a kind of *quicksilver*, a freeing of opposites, a liquidation of immobile, of previously solidified opposites.[120] This hidden fugitive quality of presence, this grayish *living silver,* could perhaps only have been discovered and turned loose with the dragonfly's assistance. Guided by its still swiftness, carried on its hermetic wings—along now with the newly released light blue of the *caelum*—it slips in through cracks opened by the violent attacks of Parkinson's disease, and the dragonfly's mercurial delight quickens immanent change.

Remembering Goethe's Mephistopheles and his introduction, "I am part of that energy that always wants to do evil, and I always end up doing good," I recall the ineluctability of Indra's Net. My Parkinson's and Mephisto surely have been in an intimately autonomous relating pattern for years. The dragonfly is often noted as being a close companion of the devil. In Germany, it is known as the devil's needle (*Teufelsnadel*), devil's bride (*Teufelsbraut*); in France, the dragonfly is the devil's agent (*Agent de diable*) to mention but a few.

The dragonfly delights in its reflection in *Faust* and flies a few dazzling darting figures in the air and then settles still on a piece of dark and fecund earth. And waits.

Neurological studies have shown that our brains have a certain plasticity. This means that this piece of biological mass can be remolded, refashioned, resculpted. My son writes me: "I read a study… if you do things habitually, Parkinson's will get in the way. If you change your habits, you ignite different parts of the brain and these parts aren't

---

[120] From Middle English quyksilver; from Old English cwicseolfor. Literally living silver from its ability to move. Perhaps like mercury (merkurius).

as impacted by Parkinson's." But what parts? I just read a short descriptive analysis of one of the latest studies of Alzheimer's and Parkinson's: "A skin test may detect Alzheimer's and Parkinson's...they both have higher levels of proteins that can be picked up in skin biopsies. That's because both skin and brain nerves start from the same tissue in the embryo." (Skin test, 2015, March 9, p. 16) Does this mean that if cells can be transplanted at the embryo stage that these two diseases can be deleted? Semantics?

No matter. Does it matter where you start...or where you—or you and it—end? Is not the process, is not the mere idea of experiencing a resculpturing of the brain alluring enough to awaken curiosity, a spirit of inquiry about change?

The centrality of me

Along with the contentious yet unwaveringly faithful accompaniment of Parkinson's, the anaclitic therapy Anna and I have been able to sustain, the faithful and loving accompaniment of Anna and of my husband, as well as the support of others, my dependence on the strength of my ego and on my will has been able to moderate its desperate urgency. I appreciate my strong will, while respecting its new ability to *dissolve in its own water*. These intimate autonomies are "the way of love" (Irigaray, 2002, p. vii).[121] I am currently feeling more balanced, healthier, and stronger than ever before.

If I have been *cast down to earth*, if my ego is not the reigning deity in the heavens any more, if the *angelic* in me has touched the *satanical* bile of Lucifer, God's fallen morning star (Isaiah 14:12), then the task remains to band together the star's illuminating brightness with the dark colors of fecund earth. Reminding myself that "every angel is

---

[121] "This book outlines...a philosophy in the feminine, where the values of intersubjectivity, of dialogue in difference, of attention to present life, in its concrete and sensible aspects, will be recognized and raised to the level of wisdom."

terrifying," I sense a space of play, as well as an imperative induction to grapple and wrestle with angels (Gen.: 28:12).

And I do not undertake this task alone. My de-light-ful constant companion, the dragonfly, suddenly reveals characteristics of both the *light-bringer*, of consciousness; and assertively it displays and narcissistically moves its intimidating and often frightening devil's needle. It darts, leaves sparks in its dusky trail, and then hides.

I have been graced by the dragonfly.

The dragonflies seem to be able to see even beyond, for they know exactly when to cease to feed before they leave the water and emerge out of their larvae. This transmutation into the adult phase is the most difficult of all. The body contracts, and wings appear. The veins, the structures hold everything together. The delicacy and the thin tissue metamorphose into a hardness that enables the dragonfly to fly. The dragonfly may not fly before drying and must sense its timing. Only then may it take off…like Rilke's angels?

For the dragonfly, the beyond is vertical as well as horizontal and is as much of a paradox as our intimate autonomy. To see a beyond conflicts with itself. I recall the philosopher maintains that a paradox "is the passion of thought, and the thinker without the paradox is like the lover without passion…." [122] The psychoanalyst knows that the paradox gradually morphs the commanding ego into an insignificant tourist. For the dragonfly and his insect brain, its passion seems to be a perpetual playing *in*—and *with* —contradictions. Its movements are not a one or the other, but both. Its relaxation is a paradigmatic example of *still dancing*, and the dragonfly's ability to see beyond is to anticipate a filled nothingness, a paradox *ipso facto*.[123]

For me, it is enough to passionately want to discover what is feels like to dare to sacrifice ego control while writing the conclusion of *The Hiss of Hope* and, instead of thinking, to let myself open to thought's thoughts. Is this paradoxical shift of subject and object an abstract

---

[122] Søren Kirkegaard.

[123] "Burnt Norton, II" is located in Appendix A-1.

strategical chess game of syntactical intellectual gymnastics? Or is it a new timid tone of the receptive passion of consciousness and creativity?

My eyes are altered now. They see differently. It's not a new landscape outside, but from behind the cataracts a new insight unfurls. An untried perspective becomes visible.

The hiss of hope (II)

Parkinson's and I have voyaged into an intimate autonomy instead of remaining stuck in a dualistic power battle. We have felt hope and at times we endured the darkness of no-hope. Somewhere along the way, however, these two opposites begin to dialogue; they begin to dance *with* each other. The choreographic sequences morph into a paradox, a relating pattern that can ultimately generate a *hiss*. This incarnation of paradox's friction is the architect of a new space. A structure giving birth. Once again, I recall my father's words: *A structure births the space and yields its predominance to its "nothingness."* The *hiss* of hope has guided Parkinson's and me into an intimately autonomous relating pattern, a pattern that for me has become the blueprint for relationships in general.

A chronic disease can devastate, destroy. But it also can open portals hitherto unknown. And then you have the opportunity to enter…Or not.

I sense and perhaps can continue *to see* beyond. I view from inside my eyes. And from behind my eyes. My quickened dragonfly brain puts tiny images together and knows moments of submission, bequeathing life, and death. And perhaps entrusts something in addition, a beyond we do not see, but one we somehow know.

An intimate autonomy, in itself, remains a paradox. Its *hiss* has no pattern or structure. It is a sound, and its space is a *nothingness*. Yet its networking weaves the world, the heavens and the earths, together. And just as Odysseus' wife, Penelope, weaves her carpet during the day and unravels it at night, *hiss* appears and disappears again and again. Life, death, love, and, above all, dialectical play, a pivotal part of the relating pattern of an intimate autonomy, are thereby summoned. I've landed in this space. Unfolding.

Without content, without thinking, yet structurally sensing a physical discernment, I let myself drift on top of the waves. Do I let myself drift? Or do the waves drift me? We are the same and not the same. The process is the process. In this intimate autonomous relating pattern with the ocean, I listen for a watery *hiss*. I feel sparks of *hope and the stings of no-hope*. I intuit the infant's need to be loved by me. A future task. Ensconced in the shifting waves and depth of oceanic waters, I drift. If I surrender to the movement, I know that I will be borne.

Freed from the opacity of ripe cataracts, I see with my new eyes not competitive antitheses of subjective thinking and objective thoughts, but rather I sense a joyful dance of opposites with twists and swirls of paradox's silvery liquidity. I do not view life and death as dissimilar, or creation and annihilation, or a life with—or without—Parkinson's disease. Instead, I feel with my new insect heart the passion and the grace of the consummation of an amazing life lived. And beyond?

Once again, I catch myself hovering. But then I suddenly recognize that I have become heavy, that I cannot just fly and float in the air. With the dragonfly an old exoskeleton is shed, and a new structure forms. Now I can sit. For hours. Doing nothing. We do wait: Parkinson's and me. I can feel the autonomy of a stillness and I can feel the intimacy of the dance. I now know the dark heaviness—of the earth and the *light*-ness of the heavens, and while I sit, I hear a swish of dragonfly wings. And these words of the poet *hiss* at me:

> You must go by way of dispossession.
> In order to arrive at what you are not
> You must go through the way in which you are not....
> And what you own is what you do not own
> And where you are is where you are not.
> (Eliot, 1941)[124]

And once again I am curious.
For the time being my voyage ends here.

March 13, 2015

---

[124] "East Coker, III," from Eliot's Four Quartets, is located in Appendix A-1.

APPENDICES

Appendix A-1: T. S. Eliot, "Burnt Norton" from The Four Quartets (1935)

Burnt Norton
(No. 1 of *Four Quartets*)

II

Garlic and sapphires in the mud
Clot the bedded axle-tree.
The trilling wire in the blood
Sings below inveterate scars
Appeasing long forgotten wars.
The dance along the artery
The circulation of the lymph
Are figured in the drift of stars
Ascend to summer in the tree
We move above the moving tree
In light upon the figured leaf
And hear upon the sodden floor
Below, the boarhound and the boar
Pursue their pattern as before
But reconciled among the stars.

At the still point of the turning world. Neither flesh nor
fleshless;
Neither from nor towards; at the still point, there the dance is,
But neither arrest nor movement. And do not call it fixity,
Where past and future are gathered. Neither movement from
nor towards,
Neither ascent nor decline. Except for the point, the still point,
There would be no dance, and there is only the dance.
I can only say, there we have been: but I cannot say where.
And I cannot say, how long, for that is to place it in time.
The inner freedom from the practical desire,
The release from action and suffering, release from the inner
And the outer compulsion, yet surrounded
By a grace of sense, a white light still and moving,
Erhebung without motion, concentration
Without elimination, both a new world
And the old made explicit, understood
In the completion of its partial ecstasy,
The resolution of its partial horror.
Yet the enchainment of past and future
Woven in the weakness of the changing body,
Protects mankind from heaven and damnation
Which flesh cannot endure.
 Time past and time future
Allow but a little consciousness.
To be conscious is not to be in time
But only in time can the moment in the rose-garden,
The moment in the arbour where the rain beat,
The moment in the draughty church at smokefall
Be remembered; involved with past and future.
Only through time time is conquered.

Appendix A-2: Hafez, "Every Child Has Known God"
Every Child Has Known God

Every child has known God,
Not the God of names,
Not the God of don'ts,
Not the God who ever does anything weird,
But the God who knows only four words
And keeps repeating them, saying:
"Come dance with Me,
come dance."

(Translated by Daniel Ladinsky)

Appendix A-3: Alfred Lord Tennyson, "The Two Voices"
The Two Voices

A still small voice spake unto me,
"Thou art so full of misery,
Were it not better not to be?"

Then to the still small voice I said;
"Let me not cast in endless shade
What is so wonderfully made."

To which the voice did urge reply;
*"To-day I saw the dragon-fly
Come from the wells where he did lie.*

*"An inner impulse rent the veil
Of his old husk: from head to tail
Came out clear plates of sapphire mail.*

"He dried his wings: like gauze they grew;
Thro' crofts and pastures wet with dew
A living flash of light he flew...."

Appendix A-4: W. H. Davies, "The Dragonfly"
The Dragonfly

Now, when my roses are half buds, half flowers,
And loveliest, *the king of flies* has come—
It was a fleeting visit, all too brief;
In three short minutes he has seen them all,
And rested, too, upon an apple tree.

There, his round shoulders humped with emeralds,
A gorgeous opal crown set on his head,
And all those shining honours to his breast—
'My garden is a lovely place' thought I,
'But is it worthy of such a guest?'

He rested there, upon the apple leaf—

'See, see,' I cried amazed, 'his opal crown,
And all those emeralds clustered around his head!'
'His breast, my dear, how lovely was his breast-'
The voice of my Beloved quickly said.

'See, see his gorgeous crown, that shines
With all those jewels bulging round its rim-'
I cried aloud at night, in broken rest.
Back came the answer quickly, in my dream-
'His breast, my dear, how lovely was his breast!'

Appendix A-5: Kahlil Gibran, "On Death"
On Death

You would know the secret of death.
But how shall you find it unless you seek it in the heart of life?
The owl whose night-bound eyes are blind unto the day
cannot unveil the mystery of light.
If you would indeed behold the spirit of death, open your heart
wide unto the body of life.
For life and death are one, even as the river and the sea are one.

In the depth of your hopes and desires lies your silent
knowledge of the beyond;
And like seeds dreaming beneath the snow your heart
dreams of spring.
Trust the dreams, for in them is hidden the gate to eternity.
Your fear of death is but the trembling of the shepherd
when he stands before the king whose hand is to be laid
upon him in honour.
Is the shepherd not joyful beneath his trembling, that he shall
wear the mark of the king?
Yet is he not more mindful of his trembling?

For what is it to die but to stand naked in the wind and
to melt into the sun?
And what is it to cease breathing, but to free the breath
from its restless tides, that it may rise and expand and seek
God unencumbered?

Only when you drink from the river of silence shall you
indeed sing.
And when you have reached the mountaintop, then you
shall begin to climb.
And when the earth shall claim your limbs, then shall you
truly dance.

Appendix A-6: Paul Celan, "Death Fugue"/"Todesfuge"
Death Fugue

Black milk of morning we drink you at dusktime
we drink you at noontime and dawntime we drink you at night
we drink and drink
we scoop out a grave in the sky where it's roomy to lie
There's a man in this house who cultivates snakes and who writes
who writes when it's nightfall nach Deutschland your golden hair
Margareta he writes it and walks from the house and the stars
all start flashing he whistles his dogs to draw near
whistles his Jews to appear starts us scooping a grave out of sand
he commands us to play for the dance

Black milk of morning we drink you at night
we drink you at dawntime and noontime we drink you at
dusktime
we drink and drink
There's a man in this house who cultivates snakes and who
writes who writes when it's nightfall nach Deutschland
your golden hair Margareta
your ashen hair Shulamite we scoop out a grave in the sky
where it's roomy to lie
He calls jab it deep in the soil you lot there you other
men sing and play
he tugs at the sword in his belt he swings it his eyes are blue
jab your spades deeper you men you other men you others
play up again for the dance

Black milk of morning we drink you at night
we drink you at noontime and dawntime we drink you at
dusktime
we drink and drink
there's a man in this house your golden hair Margareta
your ashen hair Shulamite he cultivates snakes
He calls play that death thing more sweetly Death is

a gang-boss aus Deutschland
he calls scrape that fiddle more darkly then hover like
smoke in the air
then scoop out a grave in the clouds where it's roomy to lie

Black milk of morning we drink you at night
we drink you at noontime Death is a gang-boss aus
Deutschland
we drink you at dusktime and dawntime we drink and drink
Death is a gang-boss aus Deutschland his eye is blue
he shoots you with leaden bullets his aim is true
there's a man in this house your golden hair Margareta
he sets his dogs on our trail he gives us a grave in the sky
he cultivates snakes and he dreams Death is a gang-boss aus
Deutschland

your golden hair Margareta
your ashen hair Shulamite

Todesfuge

Schwarze Milch der Frühe wir trinken sie abends
Wir trinken sie mittags und morgens wir trinken sie nachts
Wir trinken und trinken
Wir schaufeln ein Grab in den Lüften da liegt man nicht eng
Ein Mann wohnt im Haus der spielt mit den Schlangen der schreibt
Der schreibt wenn es dunkelt nach Deutschland dein
goldenes Haar Margarete
Er schreibt es und trifft vor das Haus und es blitzen die Sterne
Er pfeift seine Rüden herbei
Er pfteift seine Juden hervor lässt schaufeln ein Grab in der Erde
Er befiehlt uns spielt auf nun zum Tanz
Schwarze Milch der Frühe wir trinken sie abends
Wir trinken sie mittags und morgens wir trinken sie nachts
Wir trinken und trinken

Ein Mann wohnt im Haus der spielt mit den Schlangen der
schreibt
Der schreibt wenn es dunkelt nach Deutschland dein goldenes
Haar Margarete
Dein aschenes Haar Sulamith wir schaufeln ein Grab in den
Lüften
Da liegt man nicht eng
Er ruft stecht tiefer ins Erdreich ihr einen ihr andern singet
und spielt
Er greift nach dem Eisen im Gurt er scwingts seine Augen
sind blau
Stecht tiefer die Spaten ihr einen ihr andern spielt weiter zum
Tanz auf

Schwarze Milch der Frühe wir trinken sie abends
Wir trinken sie mittags und morgens wir trinken sie nachts
Wir trinken und trinken
Ein Mann wohnt im Haus dein goldenes Haar margarete
Dein aschenes Haar Sulamith er spielt mit den Schlangen
Er ruft spielt süsser den Tod der Tod ist ein Meister aus
Deutschland

Er ruft streicht dunkler die Geigen dann steigt ihr als Rauch
in die Luft
Dann habt ihr ein Grab in den Wolken da liegt man nicht eng
 Schwarze Milch der Frühe wir trinken sie abends
Wir trinken sie mittags und morgens wir trinken sie nachts
Wir trinken und trinken
Der Tod ist ein Meister aus Deutschland sein Auge ist blau
Er trifft dich mit bleierner Kugel er trifft dich genau
Ein Mann wohnt im Haus dein goldenes Haar Margarete
Er hetzt seine Rüden auf uns er schenkt uns ein Grab in der Luft
Er spielt mit den Schlangen und träumet der Tod ist ein Meister
aus Deutschland
dein goldenes Haar Margarete
dein aschenes Haar Sulamith

Appendix A-7 "East Coker," from *The Four Quartets* (1941)

East Coker (1941)
No. 2 of *Four Quartets*

O dark dark dark. They all go into the dark,
The vacant interstellar spaces, the vacant into the vacant,
The captains, merchant bankers, eminent men of letters,
The generous patrons of art, the statesmen and the rulers,
Distinguished civil servants, chairmen of many committees,
Industrial lords and petty contractors, all go into the dark,
And dark the Sun and Moon, and the Almanach de Gotha
And the Stock Exchange Gazette, the Directory of Directors,
And cold the sense and lost the motive of action.
And we all go with them, into the silent funeral,
Nobody's funeral, for there is no one to bury.
I said to my soul, be still, and let the dark come upon you
Which shall be the darkness of God. As, in a theatre,
The lights are extinguished, for the scene to be changed
With a hollow rumble of wings, with a movement of
darkness on darkness,
And we know that the hills and the trees, the distant panorama
And the bold imposing facade are all being rolled away—
Or as, when an underground train, in the tube, stops too
long between stations
And the conversation rises and slowly fades into silence
And you see behind every face the mental emptiness deepen
Leaving only the growing terror of nothing to think about;
Or when, under ether, the mind is conscious but conscious
of nothing—
I said to my soul, be still, and wait without hope
For hope would be hope for the wrong thing; wait without love
For love would be love of the wrong thing; there is yet faith

But the faith and the love and the hope are all in the
waiting.
Wait without thought, for you are not ready for thought:
So the darkness shall be the light, and the stillness the
dancing.
Whisper of running streams, and winter lightning.
The wild thyme unseen and the wild strawberry,
The laughter in the garden, echoed ecstasy
Not lost, but requiring, pointing to the agony
Of death and birth.

You say I am repeating
Something I have said before. I shall say it again,
Shall I say it again? In order to arrive there,
To arrive where you are, to get from where you are not,
 You must go by a way wherein there is no ecstasy.
In order to arrive at what you do not know
 You must go by a way which is the way of ignorance.
In order to possess what you do not possess
 You must go by the way of dispossession.
In order to arrive at what you are not
 You must go through the way in which you are not.
And what you do not know is the only thing you know
And what you own is what you do not own
And where you are is where you are not.

Appendix A-8: T. S. Eliot, "A Game of Chess" and "Death by Water," from The Wasteland
II A Game of Chess

"My nerves are bad to-night. Yes, bad. Stay with me.
Speak to me. Why do you never speak? Speak.
What are you thinking of? What thinking? What?
I never know what you are thinking. Think."
I think we are in rats' alley
Where the dead men lost their bones.

Part Three

IV. Death by Water

Phlebas the Phoenician, a fortnight dead,
Forgot the cry of gulls, and the deep seas swell
And the profit and loss.
A current under sea
Picked his bones in whispers. As he rose and fell
He passed the stages of his age and youth
Entering the whirlpool.
Gentile or Jew
O you who turn the wheel and look to windward,
Consider Phlebas, who was once handsome and tall as you.

Appendix A-9: Rainer Maria Rilke, Duino Elegies "The Eighth Elegy"/"Die Achte Elegie"
The Eighth Elegy

The animal that's free/
has its decline behind it always/
and before it God; and when it runs, it runs/
in eternity, the way fountains run./
(We don't ever have before us, not one single day,) the pure space into which/
flowers endlessly bloom. It is always world/
and never Nowhere without Not: (that pureness/
not watched over, that one breathes /
and endlessly knows and doesn't desire…*This is called fate:*
to be opposite/
and nothing more than opposite and always that.

Die Achte Elegie

Das freie Tier/
hat seinen Untergang stets hinter sich/
und vor sich Gott, und wenn es geht, so gehts/
in Ewigkeit, so wie die Brunnen gehen...Wir haben nie,
nicht einen einzigen Tag,/
den reinen Raum vor uns, in den die Blumen/
unendlich aufgehn. Immer ist es Welt/
und niemals Nirgends ohne Nicht...Das heisst Schicksal:
gegenueber sein/
und nichts als das und immer gegenueber

Appendix A-10: William Butler Yeats, "The Second Coming"
The Second Coming

Turning and turning in the widening gyre
The falcon cannot hear the falconer;
Things fall apart; the centre cannot hold;
Mere anarchy is loosed upon the world,
The blood-dimmed tide is loosed, and everywhere
The ceremony of innocence is drowned;
The best lack all conviction, while the worst
Are full of passionate intensity.

Surely some revelation is at hand;
Surely the Second Coming is at hand.
The Second Coming! Hardly are those words out
When a vast image out of Spiritus Mundi
Troubles my sight: somewhere in sands of the desert
A shape with lion body and the head of a man,
A gaze blank and pitiless as the sun,
Is moving its slow thighs, while all about it
Reel shadows of the indignant desert birds.

The darkness drops again; but now I know
That twenty centuries of stony sleep
Were vexed to nightmare by a rocking cradle,
And what rough beast, its hour come round at last,
Slouches towards Bethlehem to be born?

Appendix A-11: Rainer Marie Rilke, "The First Elegy"/ "Die Erste Elegie"

The First Elegy

Who, if I cried out, would hear me then, out of the orders
Of angels? And even supposing one suddenly took me
Close to the heart, I would perish from that
Stronger existence. For what strikes us as beauty is nothing
But all we can bear of a terror's beginning,
And we admire it so, because it calmly disdains
To destroy us. *Every angel strikes terror…*

Die Erste Elegie

Wer, wenn ich schreie, hoerte mich denn aus der Engel
Ordnungen? Und gesetzt selbst, naehme
einer mich ploetzlich ans Herz; ich verginge von seinem
staerkeren Dasein. Denn das Schöne ist nichts
als des Schrecklichen Anfang, den wir gerade ertragen,
und wir bewundern es so, weil, es gelassen verschmäht,
uns zu zerstören. *Ein jeder Engel ist schrecklich.*

Appendix A-12: Alfred Lord Tennyson, "In Memoriam," Section 45
In Memoriam, Section 45

The baby new to earth and sky,
What time his tender palm is prest
Against the circle of the breast,
Has never thought that "this is I":

But as he grows he gathers much,
And learns the use of "I," and "me,"
And finds "I am not what I see,
And other than the things I touch."

So rounds he to a separate mind
From whence clear memory may begin,
As thro' the frame that binds him in
His isolation grows defined.

This use may lie in blood and breath
Which else were fruitless of their due,
Had man to learn himself anew
Beyond the second birth of Death.

Appendix A-13: Rainer Maria Rilke, "Archaic Torso of Apollo" / "Archaischer Torso Apollos"
Archaic Torso of Apollo

We never knew his fantastic head,
where eyes like apples ripened. Yet
his torso, like a lamp, still glows
with his gaze which, although turned down low,
lingers and shines. Else the prow of his breast
couldn't dazzle you, nor in the slight twist
of his loins could a smile run free
through that center which held fertility.

Else this stone would stand defaced and squat
under the shoulders' diaphanous dive
and not glisten like a predator's coat;
and not from every edge explode
like starlight: for there's not one spot
that doesn't see you. You must change your life…
(My translation)

Archaischer Torso Apollos

Wir kannten nicht sein unerhörtes Haupt,
darin die Augenäpfel reiften. Aber
sein Torso glüht noch wie ein Kandelaber,
in dem sein Schauen, nur zurückgeschraubt,
sich hält und glänzt. Sonst könnte nicht der Bug
der Brust dich blenden, und im leisen Drehen
der Lenden könnte nicht ein Lächeln gehen
zu jener Mitte, die Zeugung trug.

Sonst stünde dieser Stein enstellt und kurz
unter der Shultern durchsichtigem Sturz
und flimmerte nicht so wie Raubtierfelle;

und brächte nicht aus allen seinen Rändern
aus wie ein Stern: denn da ist keine Stelle,
die dich nicht sieht. Du mußt dein Leben ändern.

Figure

The vertical and horizontal splits   254

References

Adorno, T. W. (1970). *Aesthetische theorie* [Aesthetic theory]. In G. Adorno & R. Tiedemann (Eds.), Frankfurt am Main: Suhrkamp Verlag.

Arendt, H. (1963). *Eichmann in Jerusalem*. New York: Viking Press.

Arendt, H. (1981). *The Life of the Mind*. New York: Mariner.

Armstrong, K. (2011). *Twelve Steps to a Compassionate Life*. Toronto: Vintage Canada.

Bagheri, Z. M., Wiederman, S. D, Cazzolato, B. S., Grainger, S., O'Carroll, D. C. (2015, June 10). Properties of neuronal facilitation that improve target tracking in natural pursuit simulations. *J. R. Soc. Interface 12(108)*. DOI: 10.1098/rsif.2015.0083. Retrieved April 28, 2018, from: http://rsif.royalsocietypublishing.org/content/12/108/20150083

Barrow, J. D. (2001). *The Book of Nothing: Vacuums, Voids, and the Latest Ideas About the Origins of the Universe*. New York: Pantheon.

Bartoff, H. (1996). *The Wholeness of Nature: Goethe's Way Toward a Science of Conscious Participation in Nature*. New York: Lindisfarne.

Bateson, G. (1972). *Steps to an Ecology of the Mind*. New York: Ballantine.

Becker, E. (1973). *The Denial of Death*. New York: Simon & Schuster.

Bini, J. K., Cohn, S. M., Acosta, S. M., McFarland, M. J., Muir, M. T., & Michalek, J. E. (2011, April). Mortality, Mauling, and Maiming by Vicious Dogs. *Annals of Surgery, 253*, 791-797. Retrieved April 25, 2018, from https://journals.lww.com/annalsofsurgery/Abstract/2011/04000/Mortality,_Mauling,_and_Maiming_by_Vicious_Dogs.23.aspx DOI: 10.1097/SLA.0b013e318211cd68

Bion, W. R. (1992). *Cogitations*. F. Bion (Ed.), London, UK: Karnac.

Boesel, C. & Keller, C. (Eds.). (2010). *Apophatic Bodies: Negative Theology, Incarnation, and Relationality.* New York: Fordham University.

Borchert, W. (1947). *Draussen vor der Tuer.* Hamburg: Rowohlt.

Bortoft, H. (1996). *The wholeness of nature: Goethe's way toward a science of conscious participation in nature.* Wylam, Northumberland: Lindisfarne.

Burnett, F. H. (1949). *The Secret Garden.* New York: Lippincott.

Campbell, J. (1959). *The Masks of God: Primitive Mythology.* New York: Viking.

Capra, F. (1996). *The Way of Life: A New Scientific Understanding of Living Systems.* New York: Anchor.

Caris, J. (1987). *Foundation for a New Consciousness.* San Francisco: Westgate.

Carroll, L. (1865/2009). *Alice in Wonderland.* New York: Random House.

Celan, P. (2001). Todesfuge [Death Fugue]. In *Selected Poems and Prose of Paul Celan.* (J. Felstiner, Trans.). New York: W. W. Norton.

Claudio Abbado obituary. (February 1, 2014). *The Economist.*

Das magische auge. (2002/2004). Munich: Magic Eye.

Davies, W. H. (1928). The Dragonfly. *The Dragonfly (Odonata anisoptera).* Retrieved April 30, 2018, from https://hort330-deshields.weebly.com/poem.html

Davis M. & Wallbridge, D. (1981). *Boundaries and Space: An Introduction to the Work of D. W. Winnicott.* New York: Brunner/Mazel.

De Leon, M. (2015). *Parkinson's Diva: A Woman's Guide to Parkinson's Disease.* Canton, GA: The Word Verve.

Gerald M. Edelman. (2004). *Wider Than the Sky: The Phenomenal Gift of Consciousness.* New Haven, CT: Yale University.

Edinger, E. F. (1985). *Anatomy of the Psyche: Alchemical Symbolism in Psychotherapy.* La Salle, IL: Open Court.

Edinger, E. F. (1995). *The Mysterium Lectures.* Toronto: Inner City.

Eliot, T. S. (1943). *Four Quartets.* New York: Harvest.

Isaac Newton. (1911). *The Encyclopaedia Britannica* (Vol. 19, pp. 584-585). New York: The Encyclopaedia Britannica.

Evans, R. (1964). *C. G. Jung Speaking: Interview and Encounter*. Princeton, NJ: Van Nostrand.

Fox, M. J. (2002). *Lucky Man: A Memoir*. New York: Hyperion.

Friedman, J. (August 7, 2017). It's Okay to Be a Coward About Cancer. *Time*, pp. 21-21.

Freud, S. (1914/1982). Erinnern, wiederholen und durcharbeiten [Working through repetition compulsions]. In *Schriften zur behandlungstechnik: Studienausgabe ergaenzungsband*, 207-217 *[Writings on treatment techniques: Supplementary volume for students]*. Frankfurt: Fischer Taschenbuch.

Freud, S. (1920). *Beyond the Pleasure Principle*. London: The International Psychoanalytical Press.

Ghent, E. (1983). Masochism, Submission and Surrender: Masochism as a Perversion of Surrender. *Contemporary Psychoanalysis, 26*(1), 108-136.

Gibran, K. (1932). On death. In K. Gibran, *The Prophet*. New York: Knopf.

Giegerich, W. (1998). *The Soul's Logical Life: Towards a Rigorous Notion of Psychology*. Zurich, CH: Peter Lang.

Giegerich, W. (2010). The end of meaning and the birth of man. In *The soul always thinks: Collected English papers, 4*, 189-285. New Orleans, LA: Spring Journal.

Giegerich, W. (2012). *What is soul?* New Orleans: Spring Journal.

Goethe, J. W. von. (1806/1992). *Faust: A Tragedy. Parts 1 & 2*. (M. Greenberg, Trans.). New Haven, CT: Yale University.

Goethe, J. W. von. (1821/2012). *Wilhelm Meister's Years of Travel, or, The Renunciants*. (H. M. Waidson, Trans.). London: Oneworld Classics.

Goethe, J. W. von. (1832?/1998). *Faust: A Tragedy. Part 2*. (M. Greenberg, Trans.). New Haven, CT: Yale University.

Greenberg, M. (1992). *Johann Wolfgang von Goethe, Faust: A Tragedy. Part I*. (M. Greenberg, Trans.). New Haven, CT: Yale University.

Grimm, J., Grimm, W. K. (1884/1981). *The Complete Brothers Grimm Fairy Tales*. New York: Crown.

Hafiz (13??/1999). The God Who Only Knows Four Words. In *The Gift: Poems by Hafiz, the Great Sufi Master*. (D. Ladinsky, Trans.). New York: Penguin Compass.

Heller, E. (1994). *Die wahre geschichte von allen farben* [The true story of all colors]. Oldenburg, BE: Lappen Verlag.

Hannah, B. (1981). *Encounters With the Soul: Active Imagination as Developed by C. G. Jung*. Boston, MA: Sigo.

Hauptmann, G. In *Aus Gerhart Hauptmanns diarium*. 1917-1933. (W. Stekel, Ed.). Berlin: Propylaen.

Hawkins, D. R. (1995). *Power Vs. Force: The Hidden Dimensions of Human Behavior*. New York: Hay House.

Heisenberg, W. (1967, May 21) Das naturbild Goethes und die technisch-naturwissenschaftliche Welt. Goethe-Gesellschaft, Weimar. [Lecture delivered to general assembly of Goethe-Gesellschaft, Weimar, on 21 May.]. *Jahrbuch 29*, 27-42. Source note located April 30, 2018, at: https://history.aip.org/history/exhibits/heisenberg/bibliography/1965-69.htm#1967

Hillman, J. (1979). *The Dream and the Underworld*. New York: Avon Harper and Row.

Hillman, J. (2009). Silver and the White Earth, II. In Hillman, J. *Alchemical Psychology: Uniform Edition of the Writings of James Hillman*, Vol. 5. New York: Spring.

Houlgate, S. (2015). *Introduction to Hegel: Freedom, Truth and History*. Oxford, UK: Blackwell.

Huffman, K., Younger, A. & Vanston, C. (2010). *Visualizing Psychology*. Toronto: Wiley.

Huizinga J. (1949/1955). *Homo Ludens: A Study of the Play-Element in Culture*. Boston, MA: Beacon.

Irigaray, L. (1995). *I Love to You: Sketch of a Possible Felicity*. (A. Martin, Trans.). New York: Routledge.

Irigaray, L. (2002). *The way of love*. (H. Bostic & S. Pluhàcek, Trans.). New York: Continuum.

Jones, J. W. (2002). *Terror and Transformation: The Ambiguity of Religion in Psychoanalytic Perspective*. New York: Routledge.

Josey, A. (2001). The Last Renaissance: Individuation in the Ages 70-90. *Psychological Perspectives*, *56*(2):173-183. Philadelphia, PA: Taylor and Francis.

Jung, C. G. (1961, Dec.). Interview in *Good Housekeeping Magazine*, Vol. 153, no. 6.

Jung, C. J. (1968). *Psychology and Alchemy. Collected Works: I.* (G. Adler & R. H. Hull, Trans.) Princeton, NJ: Bollingen Series, Princeton University Press.

Jung, C. G. (1971). *Alchemical studies.* (H. G. Baynes & R. F. C. Hull, Trans.). Princeton, NJ: Princeton University.

Jung, C. G. (1971). *Die psychologie der uebertragung.* Bd. 16, para. 442, Walter Verlag, Freiburg im Breisgau

Jung, C. G. (1971). *Praxis der therapie [The Fundamentals of Therapy].* Bd. 16, 178-345. Freiburg im Breisgau, DE: Walter Verlag.

Jung, C. G. (1972). *Briefe I: 1906-1945*, Bd. I. (A. Jaffe. & G. Adler, Eds.) Freiburg im Breisgau, DE: Walter Verlag.

Jung, C. G. (1973). *Briefe III 1956-1961. (Letters III).* Freiburg im Breisgau, DE: Walter Verlag.

Jung, C. G. (1982). *Studien ueber alchemistische Vorstellungen. [Fundamentals of alchemy].* Bd. 13, 211-271. Freiburg im Breisgau, DE: Walter Verlag.

Jung, C. G. (1984). *Mysterium coniunctionis,* Bd. 14/1, 62-75. Freiburg im Breisgau, DE: Walter Verlag.

Jung, C. G. (2012). *The Red Book Liber Novus.* S. Shamdasani (Ed.). New York: Philemon Series, Norton.

Kalsched, D. (1996). *The Inner World of Trauma: Archetypal Defenses of the Personal Spirit.* New York: Routledge.

Kernberg, O. (1984). *Severe Personality Disorders.* New Haven, CT: Yale University.

Kernberg, O. (1990). *Borderline Conditions and Pathological Narcissism.* London, UK: Jason Aronson.

Kierkegaard, S. (2013). *Kierkegaard's Writings, VII, Volume 7: Philosophical Fragments, or a Fragment of Philosophy/Johannes Climacus, or pe omnibus dubitandum est.* (H. V. Hong, Ed. & Trans.). Princeton University.

Kohut, H. (1971). *The Analysis of the Self: A Systematic Approach to the Psychoanalytic Treatment of Narcissistic Personality Disorders.* New York: International Universities.

Kohut, H. (1985). *Self Psychology and the Humanities.* (C. Strozier, Ed.). New York: Norton.

Lachmann, F. M. (2008). *Transforming Narcissism: Reflections on Empathy, Humor and Expectations.* New York: The Analytic.

Lahr, J. (April 12, 2010). Escape artist: Mark Rothko onstage. *The New Yorker.* (pp. 80-81). Retrieved April 30, 2018, from: https://www. newyorker.com/magazine/2010/04/12/escape-artist

Lazzarini, A. (2014). *Both Sides Now: A Journey from Researcher to Patient.* New Brunswick, NJ: Createspace Independent Publishing Platform.

Magic Eye, Inc. (2004). *The magic eye/Das magische auge.* Magic Eye: Munich, Germany.

Melville, H. (1967). *Moby Dick.* (H. Hayford & H. Parker, Eds.). New York: W. W. Norton.

Mitchell, F. L. & Lasswell J. J. (2005). *A Dazzle of Dragonflies.* College Station, TX: A&M University.

Neumann, E. (1980). *Das kind* [The Child]. Fellbach, HV: Adolf Bonz Verlag.

Oenning-Hodgson, M. (2007). The good-enough mother. In V. Bergum & J. Van der Zalm (Eds.), *Mother-life: Studies of mothering experience* (pp. 48-68). Edmonton, CA: Pedagon.

Oenning-Hodgson, M. (2009). Illness as an Illusion of Misfortune: The Hermetic Wings of the Dragonfly. *Psychological Perspectives, 2*(I), 37-54. Philadelphia: Taylor and Francis.

Okun, M. S. (2015). *10 Breakthrough Therapies for Parkinson's Disease.* Newberry, FL: Books4Patients.

Picasso, P. (1974). Statement to Marius de Zayas. (*The arts,* New York, May 1923, pp. 315-326). In A. H. Barr, Ed., *Picasso: Fifty years of his art* (pp. 270-271). Boston: Museum of Modern Art.

Pullman, P. (1995). *The Golden Compass: His Dark Materials*. New York: Alfred A. Knopf.

Raz, M. (2010). Anaclitic therapy in North America: Psychoanlytic and psychiatric practice in the 1950s–1960s. *Psychoanalysis and History 12,* 56. Jerusalem, IL: Edinburgh University.

Reynolds, R. (2018). Infidelity: The #1 Obstacle to Recovery. *Recovery Library*. Retrieved April 25, 2018, from: https://www.affairrecovery. com/newsletter/founder/infidelity-betrayal-the-number-one-obstacle-to-recovery

Rilke, R. M. (1992). *Duino elegies*. (D. Oswald, Trans.). Einsiedeln, CH: Daimon Verlag.

Robertson, R. (2009). *Indra's Net: Alchemy and Chaos Theory as Models for Transformation*. Wheaton, IL: Theosophical Publishing House.

Schenk, R. (2001). *Darklight: The Appearance of Death in Everyday Life*. Albany, NY: State University of New York.

Schenk, R. (2012). *American Soul: A Cultural Narrative*. New Orleans, LA: Spring Journal.

Seamon, D. (1978). Goethe's approach to the natural world in implications for environmental theory and education in humanistic geography prospects and problems. In D. Ley and M. Samuels (Eds.), *Humanistic geography: Prospects and problems* (pp. 238-250). Chicago: Maaroufa.

Seamon, D. (1998). *Goethe's Way of Science: A Phenomenology of Nature*. Albany, NY: State University of New York.

Seife, C. (2000). *Zero: The Biography of a Dangerous Idea*. New York: Viking.

Shadbolt, D. (1987). *The Art of Emily Carr*. Vancouver, BC: Douglas & McIntyre.

Singer, T. & Kimbles, S. L. (Eds.). (2004). *The Cultural Complex: Contemporary Jungian Perspectives on Psyche and Society*. London, UK: Brunner-Routledge.

Skin test may detect Alzheimer's and Parkinson's. (2015, March 9). *Time*, p. 16. Retrieved April 30, 2018, from: http://time.com/3721009/a-simple-skin-test-may-detect-alzheimers/

Sullivan, L. H. (1896, March). The Tall Office Building Artistically Considered. *Lippincott's Magazine 57*, 403-409. Philadelphia: J. B. Lippincott. Retrieved April 30, 2018, from: https://www.scribd.com/doc/104764188/Louis-Sullivan-The-Tall-Office-Building-Artistically-Considered

Tennyson, A. L. (2014). *In Memoriam*. Toronto: Broadview.

Tennyson, A. L. (1833). The Two Voices. Retrieved April 30, 2018, from: https://www.poemhunter.com/poem/the-two-voices-2/

Trunz, E. (1996). *Goethe–Faust* (E. Trunz, Ed.). Munich, Germany: C. H. Beck.

Von Franz, M. L. (1980). *Projection and Re-Collection in Jungian Psychology: Reflections of the soul*. (W. H. Kennedy, Trans.). London, UK: Open Court.

Waite, H. E. (1893). *The Hermetic Museum*, Vol. 1, p. 13. Retrieved April 30, 2018, from: http://www.sacred-texts.com/alc/hermmuse/index.htm

Williams, M. (1986). *The Velveteen Rabbit*. New York: Derrydale.

Winnicott, D. W. (1971). *Playing and Reality: The Use of the Object and Relating Through Identification*. New York: Routledge.

Wright, F. L. (1939). *An Organic Architecture: The Architecture of Democracy*. London, UK: Lund Humphries.

Yeats, W. B. (1921/1969). The Second Coming. In C. M. Coffin (Ed.). *The Major Poets*. New York: Harcourt, Brace and World.

About the Author

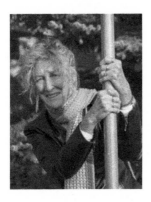

Meredith Oenning-Hodgson, originally from Colorado, is a Zurich-trained Jungian analyst. During 32 years living in Germany she developed a deep affinity for the country's culture and literature, especially Goethe. Her first Master's degree was from the University of Oregon, her second from the University of Frankfurt. She earned her diploma in Analytical Psychology from the Jung Institute, where she later became a training analyst and teacher.

After 15 years working in private practice in Frankfurt, she moved to Edmonton, Canada, where she established a Jung Forum, held weekly discussion groups, and taught at the University of Alberta. She lectured at various Canadian centers. While maintaining a full private practice, she published articles in "Psychological Perspectives" and wrote a chapter for the book *Mother Life*.

By 2008 symptoms of Parkinson's disease violently disrupted her life. *The Hiss of Hope* tells of an amazing voyage to an *intimate autonomy*, to a radically different structural pattern of relating, and to a second birth.

After a particularly cold winter, she awaits the return of the dragonflies.

CPSIA information can be obtained
at www.ICGtesting.com
Printed in the USA
FFHW022017250419
52039309-57430FF

9 781630 517007